THE CURIOUS MAN

THE LIFE AND WORKS OF DR. HANS NIEPER

HANS A. NIEPER, MD
ARTHUR D. ALEXANDER, III
G.S. EAGLE-ODEN

AVERY PUBLISHING GROUP

Garden City Park • New York

The therapeutic procedures described in this book are based on the training, personal and clinical experiences, and research of the author. They are not intended as a substitute for consulting with your physician or other health care provider. The publisher does not advocate the use of any particular treatment, but believes the information presented in this book should be available to the public. Because there is always some risk involved, the author and publisher are not responsible for any adverse effects or consequences resulting from the use of any of the suggestions, preparations, or procedures described in this book. Please do not use the book if you are unwilling to assume the risk. Feel free to consult with a physician or other qualified health professional. It is a sign of wisdom, not cowardice, to seed a second or third opinion.

Cover designer: Eric Macaluso
Cover photo: Photographie Joachim Giesel
Copyright by Alle Rechte vorbehalten
Abdruck nur gegen: Nennung
In-house editor: Helene Ciaravino
Typesetter: Elaine V. McCaw

Avery Publishing Group
120 Old Broadway
Garden City Park, NY 11040
1-800-548-5757
www.averypublishing.com

Library of Congress Cataloging-in-Publication Data

Nieper, Hans Alfred.
  The curious man: the life and works of Dr. Hans Nieper / by Hans
Alfred Nieper, Arthur Douglass Alexander, and G. S. Eagle-Oden.
    p.   cm.
  Includes bibliographical references and index.
  ISBN 0-89529-864-3
  1. Nieper, Hans Alfred.   2. Physicians—Germany—Biography.
  3. Orthomolecular therapy.   4. Cancer—Alternative treatment.
  I. Alexander, Arthur Douglass.   2. Eagle-Oden, Gene Sylvester.   3. Title.
  RM235.5.N54   1999
  610'.92—dc21
  [B]   98–46349
                                                                            CIP

Printed in the United States of America

10   9   8   7   6   5   4   3   2   1

Contents

To my wife Helga and son Daniel

and

*To all who have suffered ill-health,
having been denied access to alternative,
innovative, life-saving medical treatments.*

*A*CKNOWLEDGMENTS

Dr. Hans A. Nieper gives special acknowledgment to the following individuals, who have played important roles in his life and works:

Arthur Douglass Alexander III, biochemist and scientific consultant; former Executive Assistant to Dr. C. Chester Stock, Scientific Director of Sloan-Kettering Institute for Cancer Research (New York); a Senior Scientist in the Long Range Planning and Mission Analysis Division at NASA's Ames Research Center; and, for more than thirty years, Dr. Nieper's close friend and colleague in both cancer and space physics research.

Dr. J. Beuth, President of the German Society of Oncology.

The late Dr. Dean Burk, Head of the Cytochemistry Division, National Cancer Institute.

The late Dr. Stephen Buchner, the founder of the Freiberg University Cancer Research Laboratory.

The late Edie Goetz of Beverly Hills, California, daughter of Louis B. Mayer (MGM Studios President).

Lillian Hanke, archivist for Dr. Nieper's papers at the A. Keith Brewer International Science Library, Richland Center, Wisconsin.

Dr. F.K. Klippel, past President of the German Society of Oncology.

The late Dr. Franz Kohler, brilliant chemist; inventor of Plexiglas; and collaborator with Dr. Nieper in the synthesis of numerous important therapeutic mineral transporters and nutrient supplements.

The late Kanematsu Sugiura, DSc, senior research scientist at the Sloan-Kettering Institute who did extensive research on Laetrile.

Mrs. Monica Malchert, Dr. Nieper's staff secretary and out-patient nurse for twenty-eight years.

Dr. Ralph Moss, former Assistant Director of Public Affairs, Memorial Sloan-Kettering Cancer Center; author of ten books, including *Questioning Chemotherapy; Cancer Therapy; The Cancer Industry;* and *Free Radical;* co-producer of the PBS documentary film "The Cancer War"; foundling member of and advisor to the Office of Alternative Medicine of the National Institutes of Health.

Mrs. Susan Eagle-Oden, close friend; President and cofounder of Alpha Dependence Corporation and Nutrient Carriers, Inc., et al.—the companies in the United States and New Zealand that are exclusively licensed by Dr. Nieper to distribute worldwide his complete line of mineral trans-porters and orthomolecular and eumetabolic nutrient sup-plements.

Dr. Lloyd J. Old, MD, former Vice President of Memorial Sloan-Kettering Cancer Center.

Gene Sylvester Eagle-Oden, founder and President of the Health Freedom Foundation and the International Federation of Health Practitioner Associations. As a close friend and business associate, Mr. Eagle-Oden has helped to make Dr. Nieper's biologically oriented healthcare products available to the peoples of the world.

Ms. Christa Otto, Dr. Nieper's longtime outpatient nurse, retired in 1998.

Dr. Demetrio Sodi Pallares, friend of Dr. Nieper's since 1970; author of *Lo Que He Descubierto En El Tejido Canceroso*, a book on membrane polarization and malignant disorder.

The late Dr. Linus Pauling, Nobel Laureate in Chemistry and Nobel Peace Prize winner; proponent of orthomolecular biology in the treatment of diseases at the cellular level; strong influence on Dr. Nieper's thinking and approach to developing nontoxic cellular therapies.

Dr. C. Chester Stock, retired Scientific Director of Memorial Sloan-Kettering Cancer Center; instrumental in the design and implementation of the national chemotherapy screening program adopted by the National Cancer Institute in its search for new, effective chemotherapy (anticancer) agents.

Dr. Ernst Stuhlinger, brilliant space physicist; former assistant to Dr. Werner von Braun at NASA's Huntsville Research Center.

The late Dr. Manfred von Ardenne, brilliant medical researcher and physicist from Dresden, Germany.

𝒢OREWORD

When I arrived at Memorial Sloan-Kettering Cancer Center (MSKCC) in New York in June, 1974, there was an atmosphere of great excitement. The "war on cancer," declared by President Nixon in December, 1971, was finally gearing up. Viruses were being explored as causative agents, new chemotherapeutic drugs were being discovered, and scientific leaders, such as Robert A. Good, MD, PhD; Lloyd Old, MD; and Lewis Thomas, MD, were pioneering the immunological approach to cancer.

Yet, as I soon discovered, there was another side to the war on cancer about which few people—even those at MSKCC—knew. This involved the highly controversial "alternative" type of treatment that existed in Germany, Mexico, and even underground in the United States, itself. In the Public Affairs office, we routinely cautioned patients away from such unconventional—what we called "quack"—approaches such as Laetrile (amygdalin). Imagine how astounded I was when I discovered that Sloan-Kettering Institute's senior researcher, the late Kanematsu Sugiura, DSc, was not only conducting scrupulous research on Laetrile, but was getting positive results concerning metastases in mice.

Even more astounding was the fact that such methods, while publicly disdained by all "right-thinking" oncologists, were quietly and sympathetically being explored in private meetings on the thirteenth floor of Sloan-Kettering's Howard Building, where Drs. Good and Old had their headquarters. The person they most consulted was a youthful and obviously brilliant German doctor named Hans Nieper. In fact, it was an open secret that one of these leaders had sent his own mother to be treated by Nieper, with beneficial results. So it is not surprising that, later, many celebrities and non-celebrities would make the trek to Hannover, Germany, to be treated by Nieper.

I remember Dr. Nieper well from those days. He was a solidly built man of medium height. He had a strong, serious expression on a decidedly German face, which occasionally lit up with an almost mischievous smile. At that time, there were complaints that Dr. Nieper held the leaders of Sloan-Kettering in sway as he expounded his treatment ideas. Although Drs. Good, Old, and Thomas were world-famous immunologists, they had little practical experience in the application of alternative concepts in the treatment of cancer. In this sphere, they were pupils of Dr. Nieper.

Laetrile (amygdalin) was the focus of many discussions. Nieper, Sugiura, and the late Dean Burk, PhD, cofounder of the U.S. National Cancer Institute, revealed that Laetrile indeed had demonstrated scientific foundations. And these foundations explained Sugiura's positive test results. Nieper, in particular, carried out a fruitful exploration of the many permutations of the amygdalin molecule.

Sloan-Kettering's leaders later publicly disavowed Laetrile and denied the positive results of the research. It was a sorry moment in the history of a great institution, and a misdeed from which it is still trying to recover. Dr. Sugiura, with great courage, refused to accept distortion of his factual record. He declared, "I write what I see! Laetrile is a good palliative drug." Sugiura was hounded for doing so; I tell this story in my book *The Cancer Industry*. I, too, protested against this coverup in numerous ways, and was fired in November, 1977, for "failing to carry out [my] most basic job responsibility," which means I didn't lie when my boss told me to. However, no amount of suppression could change a single scientific fact.

The careful work of Sugiura, Burk, and, of course, Nieper continues to excite interest in the scientific world. In the 1980s, Japanese scientists discovered that benzaldehyde—a breakdown product of Laetrile—has important anticancer clinical effects. I believe that, in the end, it will be the honest scientists who will be proven right, and the knee-jerk defenders of orthodoxy who will be exposed.

Hans Nieper went on to develop a whole class of related compounds that appear to have even greater efficacy than Laetrile. In the 1970s, he worked with German chemist Dr. Franz Kohler, Sr., to design a molecule in which the l-glucose portion of Laetrile was replaced by urea. Together, they produced what are called the ureyl-, nicotinyl-, and para-aminobenzoic mandelonitriles. Even today, Nieper uses a combination of such compounds in the treatment of cancer at his Hannover clinic and at the Paracelsus Silbersee Hospital. By caving into the "quackbusters," American science has lost twenty years of the potential development of such anticancer agents.

If Hans Nieper had done only this, he would have earned a place in medical history. However, his contributions have been truly astonishing. In cancer, he is the pioneer of a whole class of gene-repairing and gene-extinguishing substances, which constitute a fresh way of looking at the cancer problem. These substances include squalene, which is shark liver oil; carnivorous plant extracts, such as carnivora; didrovaltrate, an herbal extract from the Himalayan valerian plant; acetaldehyde; benzaldehyde; DHEA; the oncostatins; and tumosteron. This excellent book will explain all of these agents and their usage, in a way that is accessible even to readers who have not had a scientific education.

Perhaps the most curious treatment from the "curious man" is the iridodials. I must admit that I laughed out loud when I first heard about these. Iridodials are derived from the bodies of ants. How much more esoteric can one get? I must say that those of us who are in the cancer field are used to the Niagara of ideas that flow from the mind of Hans Nieper. But this, I thought, really "takes the cake." Yet the more I talked to Hans about the iridodials, the more sensible and exciting this line of research appeared.

The "ant cure" is not just a fad. It brings together a number of themes that this innovative scientist has been developing for over forty years. Iridodials, Nieper explains, are a primary source of natural chemical substances called dialdehydes. These are said to be extremely powerful genetic-repair factors. Their anticancer effect was first described by Dr. Peter Thies of Hannover, Germany, in 1985, and the iridodials were first used clinically (against lung cancer) by Dr. Didier of Gifhorn, Germany. It is Hans Nieper who has made these compounds world-famous.

As Nieper explains in this book, iridomyrmex ants (much like sharks) rarely develop tumors. They are also able to host unbelievable amounts of viruses without showing any ill effects. Yet these little creatures have no immune systems! Also, their big ant colonies are found generally in areas of intense "vacuum field" energy turbulence—what Dr. Nieper calls "geopathogenic zones" or "geopathic zones." Thus, in his terms, these ants must have very strong genetic-repair systems in order to survive.

When an experienced cancer clinician tells us that he has discovered something of value, we should pay careful attention. When such a statement comes from Hans Nieper, it should make headlines. Nieper says that, in his vast clinical experience, "the iridodials outdistance most other effective substances known in the therapeutic treatment of cancer," even in terminal breast cancer cases. This is astonishing and deserves the most intense scientific scrutiny, including, in my opinion, randomized clinical trials. A key problem has been the lack of purified substance. However, as you shall learn, the ubiquitous Nieper is working on that as well.

In addition to his work on cancer, Nieper is renowned for his treatment of multiple sclerosis (MS) and other degenerative or autoimmune diseases. In fact, he was one of the early pioneers of the concept of autoimmunity. And, as if that weren't enough, he has made fundamental contributions to the physics of "vacuum field" or "zero point" energy, and even to the U.S. Star Wars program. He is a force in the study of gravity physics worldwide.

One topic that will be of special interest to Americans concerns the "Import Alert" that the Food and Drug Administration (FDA) clamped on Dr. Nieper's products in the 1980s. (See Chapter 9.) First, the FDA prohibited the free use of safe substances within our own shores, thereby forcing patients to leave the country in order to obtain their desired treatments. As these patients returned, they were treated like criminals and had their medicines confiscated at the border. Yet many of these substances were simple nutrients sold in other forms at health-food stores in the United States. Fortunately, with the passage of the new Dietary Supplement Health and Education Act of 1994, Nieper's vitamin and mineral formulas are finally available in the United States.

Today, although Americans still lack the basic health freedoms that are enjoyed by all Germans and many other Europeans, as well as the Japanese, the situation is marginally better. And one of the leading proponents of innovative medicine, Dr. Hans Alfred Nieper, continues to break new ground in research, while still caring for the patients that come to him.

—Ralph W. Moss, PhD

Dr. Ralph Moss is the Director of The Moss Reports, and the author of several books, including *Questioning Chemotherapy; The Cancer Industry;* and *Free Radical.* He also authored the award-winning PBS documentary titled "The Cancer War."

$\mathcal{P}$REFACE

After many years of urging from my patients, friends, and colleagues, I have written *The Curious Man*, an account of my life's experiences and career at the cutting edge of alternative, innovative, life-saving medicine and clinical research. I would like to provide a little background on the work that shaped this book.

I received my medical degree in Hamburg in 1952, and performed postgraduate work at some of Germany's most prestigious universities. I have conducted research at three of the world's leading cancer centers, some of which involved visiting and cooperating with the Memorial Sloan-Kettering Cancer Center in New York City. I also served as President of the German Society for Clinical Oncology for more than seven years. My work has led to regular speaking engagements at medical and scientific conferences, and I am a frequent contributor to several German scientific journals. Over the course of my career, I have published many medical and scientific papers, as well as a book on field theory physics. In fact, I formulated a "Shielding Theory of Gravity" in 1953. This theory enabled me to postulate the generation of unlimited energy from space—a phenomenon recently confirmed by leading physicists as "vacuum field" or "zero point" energy. I served as the President of the German Association of Vacuum Field Energy for sixteen years (1981 to 1997) and am now the Honorary (Past) President.

It is evident that I have spent many years in research. However, my fundamental interests have always been in clinical medicine and the welfare of individual patients. I believe that the goal of medical care is the long-term survival and well-being of the patient, not the short-term success of the treatment. I am wary of drugs and procedures that base claims merely on static measures of "tumor regression" and/or changes in laboratory values. It is true that these are important endeavors, but only if they are reflected by similarly positive changes in the patient's quality of life. A treatment is not successful if the tumor regresses but the patient is bedridden from the effects of the therapy, or if the patient dies within months from a more aggressive recurrence of cancer. Accordingly, I have always considered it my duty to provide patients with scientifically valid, nontoxic therapies that will enhance their abilities to live comfortably and productively.

Medicine has made many astonishing advances over the course of history, and the greatest strides have been made within the past couple of decades. Today, physicians successfully replace entire organs, and they routinely save the lives of patients who never would have survived in the days of Louis Pasteur or Edward Jenner. But, in making these advances, medical science has grown dangerously arrogant. It has lost touch with how much it does *not* know. In reality, despite medicine's achievements, physicians and researchers are still groping in the dark in their efforts to prevent and treat many diseases. We do not know, for example, why one person develops cancer while another does not. We do not know why one person's immune system attacks the protective coat of nerve cells, or why another's completely fails to respond to foreign invaders. We do not even know precisely how aspirin works! And while today's conventional medical science is undoubtedly built on a strong foundation, it is deprived of the light of other sciences and medical traditions.

Unfortunately, many patients in the United States are led to believe that orthodox medicine does have all the answers, and that aggressive, often toxic techniques represent the very best in medical care. Both common sense and clinical experience make it clear that this is not the case. Are not clean arteries and functional bronchi preferable to expensive heart or lung transplants? Are antibiotics that kill off healthy bacteria and leave behind stronger, more resistant pathogens really great medical advances? Is chemotherapy effective when it is more likely to kill the patient than it is to eradicate a tumor?

Faced with the limitations of medicine as it is practiced now, one would hope that physicians and researchers would look outside the current confines of modern conventional medicine for new answers. But most physicians and scientists are unwilling to accept the fact that new answers will not be found in old places. Instead, they persist in following the same pharmaceutical and chemotherapeutic paths, coming up with the same therapeutic failures.

As a young man involved in some of the earliest research on chemotherapeutic agents, many of which are still in use today, I learned firsthand how little could be gained by going down those treatment avenues. It was clear then, as it is now, that such toxic therapies do little to prolong the length and quality of patients' lives. So I looked beyond the traditional boundaries of medicine to other sciences—particularly physics, botany, and entomology (the study of insects)—for answers to the question of how best to care for my patients.

From physics, I gained a respect for the electro-chemical nature of the human body and the impact of subtle, but extremely powerful energies—including electrical and magnetic fields—on cellular function. From botany and entomology, I learned that the defense systems of seemingly primitive plants and animals have a tremendous amount to offer in the treatment of human disease. By integrating this knowledge into my day-to-day medical practice, I have been able to help my patients without subjecting them to the toxic agents that are the mainstay of so many medical treatments.

In Germany, Japan, and many other countries, the medical establishment has succeeded in balancing the need for regulations and standards with the patients' right to choose from and to have free access to all modalities of treatment. Using existing scientific knowledge and research, these nations have developed standards and guidelines for therapies that fall outside of the traditional parameters of the pharmaceutical industry. For example, treatments prescribing nutritional health-food supplements and herbal preparations are readily given. As a result, physicians in these countries can prescribe the natural agents, and patients can purchase and use them on their own with a reasonable assurance of their purity and safety. Such a system provides more options and a broader spectrum of medical treatment.

Now, after almost half of a century in the field of medicine, I am convinced of the need to let the light and air of other sciences into the edifice of modern medicine. It is time to return to the central tenet of the healer's art, "to help, or at least to do no harm." In writing this book, my own development as a scientist and physician serves as an outline for explaining a new pattern for medicine, and the accounts of my clinical and experimental experiences offer clear illustrations of its use. Whenever possible, I have presented crucial events in the order in which they occurred. However, it has been necessary to step out of this format on occasion, in order to clarify a particular scientific point. Strictly speaking, this book is not an autobiography; it is the story of what I have lived and seen to be the evolution and rise of metabolic medicine by natural selection. And simply stated, metabolic medicine works! Although I have included aspects of my personal history that have had an impact on my professional life, more detail is given to the medical breakthroughs of which I am privileged to have been a part.

$\mathcal{I}$NTRODUCTION

In January, 1964, I opened my outpatient consultation and treatment office at Sedanstrasse 21, Hannover, Germany. My late friend, the surgeon Dr. Stephan Buthner, had arranged for me to have 950-square feet of space in the doctors' building at that location. He also invited me to have inpatient hospital privileges at the Paracelsus Silbersee Clinic, which he founded in nearby Langenhagen. Thirty-four years later, I am still at the same address, but within these walls great advances in medicine have been put into practice.

With the late Dr. Franz Kohler, I developed an extensive line of inexpensive, orthomolecular substances. *Orthomolecular* refers to natural substances that work to balance the body's chemistry. Those of us in the medical field who practice orthomolecular medicine believe that it is better to use effective, natural, nontoxic substances and therapies that are less stressful to the patient and to the patient's immune system. These relatively inexpensive therapies may require months or even years of treatment to halt or reverse the disease process, but they do so without the often devastating side effects of costly toxic orthodox agents. Dr. Kohler and I came up with a collection of mineral transporters and nutritional

supplements that have proven essential to restoring cellular health and the body's natural immune system. Today,
these substances form the cornerstone of my clinical treatment of life-threatening chronic diseases.

My approaches have been successful in combating cardiovascular disease, cancer, and multiple sclerosis (MS).
Over the years, I have treated thousands of patients coming from seventy-three countries of the world—approximately 4,000 patients from North America alone. In the
United States, my work has been colored with controversy,
due to the strict regulations of the Food and Drug
Administration (FDA). But the successful results that I
have achieved with my patients speak for themselves. Let
me give you an example.

My first cancer patient, a woman who lives near Palm
Springs, California, came to me at the Silbersee Hospital near
Hannover for treatment of a progressive, non-Hodgkin's
lymphoma in the summer of 1970. She had received extensive conventional treatment in the United States, and was
finally told nothing more could be done for her . . . that she
was a "terminal" patient. I began to treat her. Over twenty-
five years later, she was still in very good shape.

The most amazing thing about this case history is that
the United States FDA confiscated shipments of her medications, which I had prescribed from the supplying pharmacy in Germany, six times over a twenty-five-year period.
Such action put her life in grave danger by leading to obvious recurrences. And six times, following release of her
medications by the FDA, fortunately, her cancer spectacu-
larly regressed. This is one case; there have been many others. Since that time, there has been a continuous migration
of many cancer patients from North America to Hannover,
seeking my cutting-edge, orthomolecular treatments.

In 1992, I attended a hearing with the FDA, at which I
met very kind people. Their response to my inquiries about
the confiscation of my patients' medications from Germany

was, "It's the law!" However, after considerable discussion, it was agreed upon that my U.S. patients can receive their medications and refills provided that their local attending U.S. physicians confirm their diagnoses and also the unavailability of these medications in the United States. This has worked out very well. In fact, some of these FDA officials, especially those in peripheral posts, have actually referred cancer and MS patients to me.

So now that the knowledge and the treatments are available, it is time for you to learn about the strides being made when it comes to treating many of today's most threatening diseases. I want to share my work and success with you so that you can be an informed healthcare consumer and receive the best of medicine, if need be. Throughout the chapters of this text, you will learn of the various alternative methods that my colleagues and I have developed and made available. You will learn about what is not readily discussed and promoted in the American healthcare system. The goal of my book is to bring you hope in and greater knowledge about your healthcare options, as well as greater confidence in what can generally be called medical science.

CHAPTER 1

$\mathcal{C}$HILDHOOD AND THE WAR

If I were summing up the qualities of a good teacher of medicine, I would enumerate human sympathy, moral and intellectual integrity, enthusiasm, and ability to communicate, in addition, of course, to knowledge of his subject.

—Dr. Hans A. Nieper (b. 1928)

Like many doctors, my interest in medicine began long before my actual medical career. As the child (and grandchild) of physicians, medicine has been a part of my life for as long as I can remember. There was never really any doubt that, one day, I would become a doctor. With the exception of a brief period of time in which I wanted to be a forest ranger, I have always known that my place is in the field of medicine.

Throughout my childhood, I was intrigued and encouraged by medical and scientific questioning. My family name, loosely translated from German, means "the curious man." It is an apt description not only of me, but also of my parents, Drs. Margarete and Ferdinand Nieper. Of the many scientists who have taught me over the years, they were my first and best teachers.

MY FAMILY

My father was the grandson of Dr. Ferdinand Wahrendorff, founder of the Wahrendorff Psychiatric Hospitals, and son of Dr. Herbert Nieper, one of the most reputed surgeons of his time. Grandfather Nieper served as Chief Surgeon at the hospital in Goslar, Germany, where he performed the first partial resection of the stomach in 1876. The clinical complex in Goslar is named the "Dr. Herbert Nieper Hospital," and remains a part of the Gottingen University Hospital.

The Wahrendorff Hospitals, located only a few kilometers from the City of Hannover in the town of Ilten, were both the family business and the family home for three generations. When my great-grandfather established the Hospitals, he went against all the prevailing wisdom concerning the treatment of the mentally ill. Instead of merely warehousing or medicating patients, the Hospitals encouraged patients to work and to maintain some sense of autonomy and dignity. The brick buildings were designed to allow the free flow of light and air. Broad lawns and carefully tended gardens separated the wards and administrative buildings, and large trees shaded the connecting walkways. It was an unusual, even revolutionary, sanitarium. And it became the largest and most successful private facility in Europe.

When my father was born in 1887, my grandparents named him after his grandfather, Ferdinand. Like his namesake, my father had a quick mind and an insatiable scientific curiosity. Although he eventually specialized in psychiatry and neurology, my father spent several years in pharmaceutical research and was also a surgeon, technical engineer, and architect. He found a woman with an intellect that equaled his own in my mother, Margarete Krauss.

Compared to my father's family, which had been in Hannover since the thirteenth century, my mother's family was relatively new to Germany. Her maternal grandparents, the Mayer-Seramins, came to Hannover from northern Italy in the mid-1800s, in part because of Germany's well-known tolerance toward people of Jewish descent. Like their paternal grandparents, the Krauss', the members of the Mayer-Seramin clan were business people with a flair for invention and entrepreneurship. My great-great-great-grandfather became a family legend after developing the first shoe polish that could be applied to a shoe and then buffed to a shine.

Surrounded as she was by business people and inventors, it may seem strange that my mother found her way into the field of medicine. But in addition to her bright and extremely supportive family, my mother was greatly influenced by her godfather, Eugen Fischer, Director of the world-renowned Kaiser Wilhelm Institute in Berlin. By the time she met my father in late 1922, my mother had already established herself as a neurologist and psychiatrist.

My parents met when both were assistant doctors (the equivalent of residents) at a municipal hospital on the shores of Lake Constance. They married in 1925, after an eighteen-month courtship. Shortly after their wedding, my parents joined the staff of the Wahrendorff Hospitals. The isolated life in Ilten suited them well. Despite their brilliance, they were very shy, feeling uneasy outside of their immediate circle of friends and the community of medical and scientific researchers. In the comfortable yet intellectually stimulating environment of the Hospitals, my parents could satisfy their thirst for knowledge without straying too far from home. This was the world into which I was born on May 23, 1928, when my mother was thirty years old, and my father was forty-one years old.

THE YOUNGER YEARS

The sprawling grounds of the Wahrendorff Psychiatric Hospitals were an ideal environment for a growing boy. The shade trees and garden were a perfect setting for playing "cowboys and Indians" with my friends, and as the only child of the hospital's senior doctor, I was granted an almost idyllic freedom. Even more important than physical freedom, however, was the abundant intellectual freedom that my parents granted me. The love of scientific debate permeated their lives, and I was usually present at the lively discussions between my parents and their various colleagues.

So from almost before I could talk, I was surrounded by stimulating conversations about the nature of the mind, the relationship between biology and mentality, and the validity of orthodox medicine. As I matured, I was encouraged to join in these debates, asking questions and raising points of my own. Not everyone agreed with this policy. When I was five or six, an elderly relative complained to my mother, "Hans is like a little dachshund, always with his nose into things." Although I doubt it was meant as a compliment, my mother quickly appropriated the phrase and began referring to me as her "little dachshund."

In 1932, when I was a little more than four years old, a young woman was transferred to the Wahrendorff Hospitals from a hospital in Berlin. Though accompanied by a nurse, her papers and records were not with her, and there was some confusion concerning her identity and diagnosis. As senior physician, my father was the first to interview the patient. It was one of the most surprising diagnostic interviews of his professional life.

The patient who had been transferred to his care said she was the Grand Duchess Anastasia, the only surviving child of the last Czar of Russia! The woman, who was known as Anna Anderson, stayed at Wahrendorff for approximately eighteen months, and remained in contact with my father for a year or so following her release. During her time at the Hospitals, my father and his colleagues became convinced that "Anna Anderson's" claims were true, that she had survived the slaughter of her father Czar Nicholas, her mother, a brother, and three sisters.

For my part, I remember Anastasia as a pretty lady with wide-set blue eyes and a full mouth, who was always very kind to me. I quickly got into the habit of visiting with Anastasia on the balcony of her room. While overlooking the gardens, Anastasia would teach me English phrases and listen to my childish stories. I so enjoyed our time together. When Anastasia left the Wahrendorff Hospitals in the summer of 1933, my parents maintained their interest in her case and followed the news accounts of her battle for recognition. Throughout, they believed that the young woman for whom they had cared was the Grand Duchess Anastasia; I, too, had no doubts about the identity of my pretty English tutor. My father collected extensive research, but it was lost in March, 1945, due to a bomb. Yet the evidence has been confirmed by more recent documentation that suggests there is no question about "Anna's" true identity as Anastasia.

While growing up at Ilten, I was taught to think analytically, to question orthodox assumptions, and to explore my ideas and thoughts without fear of censure or ridicule. I was also largely insulated from life beyond the confines of the Institute. My parents' protection gave me the freedom to follow my dreams without being confronted with the more sober realities of life. However, my curiosity and urge for experiencing the realities of the outside world soon became motivating factors in shaping the future direction of my life.

THE WAR YEARS

I was just short of five years old when, in January of 1933, the Third Reich emerged as the dominant political force in

Medicine and the Third Reich

Although the rise of the National Socialists made barely a ripple in my young life, their medical policies had a profound impact on my parents. At first, Ferdinand and Margarete Nieper, like many German physicians, must have greeted the new regime with a certain degree of hope. The chaos of the Weimar Republic left deep scars on the medical profession, and many German doctors hoped that the new government would remedy the problems. Whatever my parents' private hopes, however, it could not have been long before they became concerned about the changes in their profession and in their nation.

In 1933, the National Socialist German Workers Party (NSDAP) publicly declared its intention to phase out all female doctors from the German medical community. The policy was based on the *volkisch* (folk; traditional populist) dogma that women should marry, stay at home, and bear children. Although little action was taken, government endorsement of this dogma nevertheless sent a very clear message to physicians such as Margarete, my mother. Female doctors were not welcome in the Third Reich. Over time, it became obvious that specialists—particularly specialists in "marginal" fields such as psychiatry—would also be less than welcome, as the Reich placed greater and greater emphasis on general practitioners.

The passage of the Nuremberg race laws in September of 1935 further communicated the Reich's definition of who was acceptable to the New Order. These detailed and restrictive laws could not help but cause my parents alarm. According to the new law, in order to retain Reich citizenship, all Germans had to be able to prove a predominantly Aryan background. While this posed no problem for my father and I, it was remotely possible that my mother, who had one Jewish grandparent and was also a female physician in an unpopular specialty, could be singled out.

Matters became more serious in December of 1935, with the establishment of the Reich Physicians' Ordinance. The Ordinance established codes of professional conduct for all who were practicing medicine within the Reich. Among these codes was a requirement that all physicians report to the authorities any and all serious cases of alcoholism, "imbecilism," and hereditary or congenital illnesses.

My parents managed to shield me from their concerns during these years, but the changes in the rules governing their profession cut perilously close to home. The Reich's new doctrines went against much of what my family held dear about medicine, science, and their country. The safe haven of the sanitarium at Ilten did not remain a safe haven for long.

Germany. The Third Reich actually came to power by popular demand (election), a fact often overlooked by many. Strange though it may seem, the rise of the National Socialist Party made little difference in my childhood. I continued to play with the same group of children; I continued to see the same pediatrician—a Jewish colleague of my father; I continued to listen eagerly to my parents' scientific debates.

I felt the first winds of change in 1938, the year in which my mother stopped practicing medicine and my father left the Wahrendorff Psychiatric Hospitals. In retrospect, I now believe it was a preemptive maneuver on his part. The Reich's attitude toward psychiatric patients was disturbingly evident. Indeed, the government-mandated euthanasia program of eliminating "defective" persons was only a year away. War looked inevitable and, though only fifty-one years of age, my father was not likely to be drafted. He must have known that he and his family would be more secure if he was not affiliated with a private, specialized psychiatric hospital. When war was declared in September of 1939, my father was already established in a new practice. He spent the war years working in a military hospital in Hannover, monitoring the health status of railroad workers.

My next brush with the realities of National Socialism came in the fall of 1940, when I was sent to spend several months with my aunt in Freiburg, not far from the French border, because of the increasing frequency of British air raids on Hannover. An old, beautiful city near the Black Forest, Freiburg was one of my favorite places, and I relished any opportunity to spend time with my aunt. At this time, I was only twelve years old, and still far more interested in science fiction and Westerns than the war and current events. My ever-protective parents did nothing to discourage this political apathy. Although I knew that my pediatrician had moved to the United States, and was vaguely aware of the violence elsewhere in Germany, it was not until my trip to Freiburg that I really became aware of the actions being taken against German Jews.

I returned home one afternoon to find my aunt standing outside, her hands tightly clenched, her face troubled. One of the neighbors—a kind, older Jewish lady by the name of Mrs. Fliess—was being taken away by two men. Confused, I ran to her and asked where she was going. After a quick glance at the men, Mrs. Fliess hugged me, told me to be a good boy, and turned away as she was put into a black car, which quickly sped away. Later, when I pressed my aunt for more information, she said that the government had been deporting many Jewish people, and that Mrs. Fliess was probably being taken to a detention camp in Alsace, on the other side of the Rhine. My aunt's guess was tragically correct. At the end of the war, we attempted to find Mrs. Fliess and learned that she had died in a camp in the Pyrenees, along with thousands of other German Jews who were deported that fall.

My parents and I continued to make Ilten our permanent residence until late 1942, when the Director of the Wahrendorff Psychiatric Hospitals informed my parents that they could no longer live in staff housing. Since my father was working increasingly long hours, my parents decided to move into Hannover to be closer to the hospital. The shift from rural Ilten to the urban center of Hannover was a shock. Although only a few kilometers from Ilten, the war was a much more real and present threat in Hannover, a major industrial city with hundreds of potential targets for Allied bombers. Air raids were a regular event; my parents and I soon became used to retreating to a neighbor's cellar when the sirens sounded. My parents' presence and constant reassurance kept me calm and gave me a feeling of security, though it was a very frightening experience for me, as it must have been for everyone involved.

School in Hannover also was much different from my school in the quiet railroad junction of Lehrte, near Ilten. At Lehrte, my teachers had shown little interest in promoting National Socialist propaganda. In Hannover, such indoctrination was standard fare. However, the war was not going well, so pressuring the "new boy" to join the Hitler Youth was not a big priority. I was able to evade what little pressures there were simply by keeping to myself—an easy task in a new environment.

In addition to the greater focus on National Socialist propaganda, the curriculum in Hannover was much more difficult. At first, I did quite poorly in mathematics, chemistry, and physics. Then, one of my parents' colleagues advised them to give me phosphate salts and, within eight weeks, my grades skyrocketed. This experience would have important ramifications on my work on mineral transporters, many years later.

I did not have much time to enjoy my new success or to become completely comfortable in my new surroundings. The fortunes of war were turning, and as more and more German soldiers were killed or taken prisoner by the Allies, all branches of the military became desperate for men. In January of 1944, my male classmates and I were drafted into the German Air Force. I was sixteen years old.

After a very short training period, I found myself back in Freiburg, where my friends and I were scattered around the city's airport, crouched behind anti-aircraft guns, scanning the skies for Allied planes. My feelings about this experience were mixed. After so many years in the secluded world of Ilten and the Wahrendorff Psychiatric Hospitals, my sudden involvement in the war was both scary and exciting. At times, as we sat behind our guns, occasionally talking in hushed tones on our phones, it felt like one of the games I had played among the trees at Wahrendorff. But when the sirens blasted, the searchlights began crisscrossing the skies, and the voices on the phones became strained and frightened, any illusion that it was all a game was stripped away. We had to fight off more than a dozen attacks of American P-47 Thunderbolt fighters. Miraculously, there were no losses on our side.

Freiburg was a small city with a comparatively small industrial base. Nevertheless, it was a primary target for the bombers sweeping into Germany. Although many of Freiburg's older buildings were destroyed during the war, the town was spared the damage that was common in Hannover, where British and American planes were pounding industrial and military targets around the entire city. In Hannover, local hospitals were often hard-pressed to care for the casualties, since medical personnel and supplies were running short. As I searched the skies above Freiburg, my father worked nearly round-the-clock in Hannover.

In the middle of March, word spread that the Allies were approaching from all sides. For Germany, the war was clearly over. On March 21, 1945, still at sixteen years of age, I was permitted to leave Freiburg and headed north through the rapidly narrowing corridor between the advancing Russian and American armies. I had not seen my parents for months. I wanted to go home.

Throughout most of the war, my family had been very lucky. The house we had rented in Hannover was untouched, my parents had suffered no injuries during the intense bombing raids on Hannover, and I had been sent to a relatively safe location when I was drafted. On March 28, 1945, as I rushed to Hannover, our luck ran out.

I arrived at our home three days after an air raid. There, I found a huge bomb crater and a pile of rubble where our house had been. I was terrified, experiencing pure panic and loss. Had my parents been killed? To my great relief and joy, I soon learned that my mother and father were alive and unharmed. Fortunately, my father had been at work in the military hospital and my mother was in a neighbor's basement when our rented home was hit by one of the last bombs to fall on Hannover. All of our belongings were destroyed, leaving my parents with the clothes on their backs and what little else they could salvage from the wreckage.

THE ALLIED OCCUPATION

On April 4, 1945, a few days after my return to Hannover, victorious United States troops marched into the city. The majority of the soldiers were Texans from in and around

Dallas. To me and my young friends, the Texans were a unique experience: generous, boisterous, with accents that we thought only existed in cowboy movies. Many were also immensely kind.

Like most of Germany, Hannover was in chaos at the end of the war. An enormous number of buildings—both residential and industrial—were in ruins, and the war had wreaked havoc on the food production and distribution. My parents and I were fairly comfortable living with family members, but many others were dependent on the aid of the occupying forces for their food and shelter.

The American troops did what they could to help regular citizens recover from the war, offering assistance whenever there was need. For instance, not long after the Americans arrived, I became very ill with acute appendicitis. Although the hospital was functioning, there was a critical shortage of ambulances, and my parents had no idea how they were going to get me to the hospital for an emergency appendectomy. In an act that was typical of the kindness of the occupying troops, an American soldier transported me there in a captured Wehrmacht (military) automobile.

When Germany officially surrendered, the country was partitioned among the four Allied nations. Hannover came under the control of the British, who soon replaced the Americans. The British, like the Americans, were also kind to the people of Hannover and did their best to help the many who were in desperate straits after the war. Slowly, but steadily, order was restored, and I was able to reestablish myself on the path toward becoming a physician.

CHAPTER 2

MEDICINE MEETS PHYSICS

There is no art which may not contribute somewhat to the improvement of medicine, nor is there any one which requires more assistance . . . from every other science.

from "A Discourse Upon the Institution
of Medical Schools in America"
—John Morgan (1735–1789)

After months as a "Waffen helper" (homeguard) during World War II, and after the tense journey back to my destroyed home, I was grateful for order and had only one desire—to resume my education. At seventeen years of age, I had already been through two schools, one war, and a foreign occupation. I had had enough adventure. I wanted to return to my studies for a career in medicine.

Picking up where life before World War II had left off was more easily said than done. In addition to the problem of inadequate and damaged facilities, there was the much deeper problem of faculties and curricula that had been adapted to fit

Nazi ideology. The Allied military authorities made rehabili-
tating the educational system one of their first priorities,
screening teachers for "political reliability," restoring damaged buildings, and printing new textbooks. Thanks to these
efforts, ten of Germany's twenty-five universities had reopened by the fall of 1945. But space was still terribly limited. I had to wait to resume my studies until the autumn of
1946, when the French opened a long-dormant university at
Mainz.

STUDYING AT MAINZ

Mainz had been without a major university for 130 years.
Although Mainz itself is quite old—it was a Celtic set-
tlement before the Romans built a town there in the first
century B.C.—the newly reopened Johann Gutenberg
University was very modern. Classes were held in a former
anti-aircraft artillery barracks—an enormous building with
tremendous installations and big assembly halls. I was
among the first class of students to enter Johann Gutenberg
University in the fall of 1946.

As a physician with a clean war record, my father had no
difficulty getting work, so affording the university was not
a problem for me. Food, however, was often in short supply. So it was a surprise when, soon after my arrival at
Mainz, my aunt sent me a parcel of food. It was not until
then that I learned the full details of my family's activities
during the Third Reich.

Although it was not explained to me at the time, my
pediatrician's "move" to the United States actually had
been a carefully planned escape, orchestrated in part by
my father. In addition, my father and several of his
coworkers had conspired to hide a Jewish colleague from
the Nazis for the entire length of the war. My uncle in
Frankfurt also took valiant measures, helping more than a
dozen of his Jewish friends and colleagues to get out of

Germany between 1933 and 1940. During the difficult years immediately after the war, these friends did their best to help my family by sending food, clothing, and other supplies whenever they were able. Years later, these same friends would further contribute to my career endeavors in a very special way.

The program at Mainz was the equivalent of an American undergraduate program, with preclinical studies in anatomy, physiology, chemistry, and the basic sciences. Despite the large size of the lecture halls, classes were often crowded, with more than 150 students at a single session. Sometimes it took careful planning just to secure a decent seat at the more popular lectures. There was one particular chemistry course for which competition was especially fierce. I realized that the best way to guarantee a good seat was to sign up for a class immediately preceding one of the two chemistry lecture sessions. I had two choices: debt law or physics. I chose physics, and it turned out to be one of the most significant decisions of my life.

Coincidentally, in 1946, physics became one of the most active areas of scientific research in the world. The year before, the United States had unleashed the power of the atom bomb, putting an end to the Pacific war and launching the nuclear age. It was, to borrow an Americanism, "a whole new ballgame," and physics was the star player.

Much of the basic science curriculum at Mainz proved to be a real disappointment. Instead of the dynamic exchange of ideas to which I had grown accustomed between my parents and their colleagues at Ilten, many of my classes were but a mechanistic presentation of facts that required little more than a fast pen and a good memory. My childhood experience at the Wahrendorff Psychiatric Hospitals had been an intellectual utopia by comparison.

However, I did find my classes in physics immensely exciting. In fact, during physics class, I felt like I was back at Ilten. Our instructor, Professor Klumb, had a love of

The Shielding Theory
of Gravity

From the time of Newton onward, the term *aether* was applied to the "cosmic sea" through which light and the forces of gravity, electricity, and magnetism travel like waves across the earth's oceans. Implicit in these early views was the assumption that the aether had a *physical* reality. Accordingly, many early physicists sought to prove the aether's physical existence.

Einstein defined "relativity" as $E=mc^2$: mass (m), when traveling at the speed of light (c) times itself (c^2), is converted into total energy. (To give you an idea of how powerful total energy is, consider the fact that an atom bomb actually only converts about 3 to 5 percent of its mass into energy!) In the wake of the success of the relativity theory, Einstein, like many other physicists, struggled with the perennial problem of developing a unified field theory that would account for electricity, magnetism, *and* gravity. He was unsuccessful, and his failure apparently caused him to have doubts of his own, concerning the ultimate fate of relativity. In 1948, Einstein wrote to his good friend, Maurice Solovine, "You seem to think that I look back upon my life's work with serene satisfaction. Viewed more closely, however, things are not so bright. There is not an idea of which I can be certain. I am not even sure I am on the right road."

Many things changed in the course of the twentieth century. The discovery of microwaves, radiation, and other forces showed that the supposed vacuum (emptiness) of space is actually teeming with energy.

Even the once-unquestioned principle of a constant "speed-of-light"—one of the cornerstones of relativity theory—has been challenged. It should not be surprising, then, that some of the finest minds in theoretical physics have revived the concept of the aether as not only a physical entity, but as a *sea of limitless energy.*

At the age of nineteen, I became very interested in this great source of energy and began to probe into concepts of gravitational force. Listening to Professor Klumb's lectures on physics at Johann Gutenberg University, I began to have severe doubts about the prevailing theories of gravitational acceleration. In particular, I could not understand how a gravitational force of "attraction" could explain this acceleration. I reasoned that the energies involved in gravitational acceleration had to be an extremely powerful radiation that causes an absorptive loss of energy in the bodies it penetrates and *pushes* the objects to gravitate (to move under the influence of gravity), as opposed to *pulling* them, as was classically theorized. Of all the great physicists, only Isaac Newton kept this option open. All of the other gravity theories, especially that of Albert Einstein, could not convince me otherwise.

In 1970, I discussed my hypothesis with Dr. Stokes of Telluron in Santa Monica, California. It was he who supported me and created the phrase "Shielding Theory of Gravity." In 1972, I wrote a letter to Dr. Ernest Stuhlinger, space physicist with Dr. Werner von Braun in Huntsville, Alabama. Stuhlinger strongly supported my hypothesis and commented that Dr. Gerald Feinberg at Columbia

University in New York had come up with a "faster-than-light" *tachyon* radiation theory. Dr. Stuhlinger subsequently wrote to me that Feinberg's hypothesis would support a Shielding Theory of Gravity.

About this same time, a document describing the "Magyary Phenomenon" came into my hands. Professor Magyary in Hungary had discovered that "At the peak of a solar eclipse, when the Moon is between the Sun and our Earth, the Sun takes away from the Moon a portion of its normal mass effect on the Earth." According to Newton and Einstein, the gravitational acceleration towards the moon should have been increased; instead, it was actually decreased. The Shielding Theory of Gravity is the only theory that can explain this finding. In a short lecture at NASA's Ames Research Center in California in March 1977, I explained how the "Magyary Phenomenon" can be explained. Later, my Shielding Theory evolved into the "Perisolar Cushion Field Theory."

Since the 1970s, assumptions of tremendously energetic fields throughout space and our universe have very solidly underscored my concept of the Shielding Theory of Gravity, which is now supported by a number of experimental proofs. Important physicists like Drs. Magyary, Mead, Hassel, and Puthoff agree with me that gravitational forces might be *absorptive* in character, as Magyary initially suggested. I have written and/or edited over 8,000 pages on the Shielding Theory of Gravity, which are available through the A. Keith Brewer International Science Library in Richland Center, Wisconsin. (See the Suggested Readings list, page 177, for more information.)

In 1994, the argument for the aether was greatly strengthened when a paper entitled "Beyond $E=mc^2$" appeared in *The Sciences*. In it, three eminent physicists—Bernard Haisch, Alfonso Rueda, and Harold Puthoff—presented a radically different interpretation of Einstein's revolutionary formula. Instead of being an expression of "the conversion of one fundamental thing, mass, into another fundamental thing, energy," these scientists suggested that $E=mc^2$ is, in fact, "a statement about how much energy is required to give the appearance of a certain amount of mass" (emphasis added). Like Tesla and other proponents of the aether, Haisch, Rueda, and Puthoff postulate that all forms of energy—including gravity, inertia, and even mass itself—arise from a vast, all-pervasive field of energy dubbed the *zero point field* or *ZPF*. (ZPF exists even at absolute zero temperature [-273°F]—hence, the name.) If they are correct, and a growing body of evidence indicates they may well be, the day may not be far off when we, as Nikola Tesla predicted, access "a limitless power obtainable everywhere in the universe and harness the very wheelwork of nature."

I have no doubt that the tremendous energies stored in the vacuum space field can be converted or harnessed into usable forms of energy. Events are happening that will require that we accomplish this great task in the near future. For example, the new German government has ruled the ending of nuclear energy. Vacuum field energy conversion is the only reasonable alternative to nuclear and hydrocarbon energy.

physics that rivaled my parents' love of medicine. He saw physics as a tool for investigating all of the fundamental rules of the universe, and defined it as "the universal science relating all energy and matter."

I also remember the warm smile and challenging lectures of my undergraduate professor of inorganic chemistry and clinical physics at Mainz—the world-renowned Fritz Strassmann. In 1938, only eight years prior, Strassmann and his colleague Otto Hahn had performed the first nuclear fission. Just after the war, the French built an important nuclear institute for Strassmann, which the undergraduates were unfortunately not permitted to enter.

Unlike anatomy, or even chemistry, whose basic principles have not changed appreciably in centuries, physics is a vital, evolving science in which new models, hypotheses, and axioms are continually being formulated. In physics, a wide range of theories not only coexist, but thrive. By examining nature from many different perspectives, physics has yielded some of the most exciting scientific developments of the twentieth century, and almost always on the basis of theories that would never survive within the more rigid constructs of medicine.

As a premedical student, I was eager to apply the tools of physics to the study and practice of medicine. In addition to my required reading, I sought out the works of Einstein and other theoretical physicists, including Nikola Tesla, Paul Dirac, Peter Higgs, and Richard Feynman. Their research and theories pointed to the tantalizing possibility that gravity, electricity, and magnetism are all manifestations of a single, immensely powerful energy field that pervades all space in the universe. Unlike the static "aether" concept of traditional physics, this "vacuum field" is highly energetic and is both the source and final destination of all forms of energy. (See "The Shielding Theory of Gravity," page 20.) Later, I realized that the existence of such a field, with all of its pervasive energy, has critical implications for the practice of medicine. The more I read about this subject, the more convinced I became that medicine had no future if it did not recognize the energetic functions of the human body, and the powerful influence of the so-called "vacuum field."

RESEARCHING THE VACUUM FIELD'S EFFECT ON THE BODY'S CELLS

Over the course of my studies in medicine and physics, both at Mainz and afterward, I came to the startling realization that the spark of life could be traced to the energy of the vacuum field. Contrary to traditional medical belief, the electrical charge of the cell membrane is not intrinsic to the membrane itself; *it is derived from the energetic vacuum field.* Cellular membranes, whose main field strength is about 90 kilovolts (kv) per centimeter, merely "condense" or absorb the energy of the vacuum, concentrating it into their complex structures and using it to maintain normal life functions. The integrity of this condenser function determines the quality of life. When it is compromised beyond repair, the spark (charge) of life literally goes out.

I believe the interaction of living cells and the vacuum field may already have been demonstrated on film. In Kirlian photographs, living matter is shown to have an energetic aura that can be captured on film by applying a very high-voltage, low-amperage field toward an organic object. More significant, however, is a "phantom" effect that occurs when, for example, the tip of a leaf is cut off before the leaf is placed on the photographic plate. After the high-voltage field is applied, the photographic plate reveals the leaf's aura, a "flare" along the cut line, and, most dramatically, a phantom image of the missing portion of the leaf! This phenomenon seems to indicate that living cells radiate energy into the vacuum, and that the field retains the "impression" of that matter and living energy.

The importance of electricity to the proper functioning

of the body—particularly of the heart—has been known almost since the dawn of medical science. There are records of physicians in ancient Greece using the electrical current produced by some species of stingrays to restart hearts. Centuries later, modern physicians use electrical paddles to do precisely the same thing.

We now have machines that can chart the electrical activity of the heart, muscles, nerves, and brain. Modern medicine routinely defines life by the presence of an electrical potential, and death by its absence. A patient is not considered truly dead until there is no evidence of electrical activity in the heart and the brain. For the purpose of science and medicine, electricity is the spark of life. Yet, despite the development of increasingly sophisticated diagnostic and monitoring devices for measuring the electrical activity of the body, medicine has never questioned the source of this enormous energy, or why it eventually fades. Furthermore, medicine has largely neglected the therapeutic implications of this electrical activity and availability.

This realization had a profound effect on my understanding of disease processes. Like all good medical students, I already knew that normal cellular functions depend on the maintenance of a very precise electrical balance within and without the cell, and that relatively minor changes in that balance can have catastrophic consequences. For example, people die from classic diarrheal diseases, such as cholera, not just because they lose fluid, but because they lose *electrolytes*—electrically charged particles that come from dissolved salt—which leads to potentially fatal disruptions in nerve and muscle function. But the addition of the energy field to this picture unveiled an entirely new dimension to the possible causes and treatments of disease.

Just as relatively minor changes in the composition of the atmosphere have a major effect on respiration (ask anyone who has gone hiking in the oxygen-thin air of the

Rockies or the Alps), so changes in the vacuum field, such as the presence of electrical or magnetic fields, have profound effects on cells. Constant exposure to even a low-level electrical or magnetic field can cause enough of a disruption to alter cellular messages, disable normal repair mechanisms, or even change the expression of reproductive genes.

In the late 1940s, when I first became aware of the importance of the vacuum field to medicine, DNA had yet to be discovered. My speculations were based purely on logic and intuition (the tools of physics!). Since then, researchers from around the world have confirmed many of my hypotheses, demonstrating that electromagnetic fields have a tremendous effect on cellular function and that these effects are involved in a wide range of disease processes.

Some very fine research has been done concerning the impact of electromagnetic fields on human cells, including important studies by W. Ross Adey of Loma Linda University in California; Hans Wieser of the University Hospital in Zurich; Michael Fuller of the University of California at Santa Barbara; and Jon Paul Dobson of the Swiss Federal Institute of Technology. All of these researchers have shown, beyond a shadow of a doubt, that living cells do respond to energetic fields, and that the presence of some forms of energy can drastically alter cellular function. When coupled with other risk factors, such as poor diet, exposure to toxic chemicals and other carcinogens, and a sedentary lifestyle, constant exposure to certain types of energetic fields can pave the way for cancer, heart disease, and even autoimmune disorders. But there is also a heartening side to this story. Humans are living conduits of (and exist because of) the energy of the universe. This fact carries with it the possibility that we can learn to actively *control* this energy and use it in positive ways.

My full appreciation of the importance of the vacuum field would not come until many years after I left Johann Gutenberg University. But my three years of preclinical studies and the wonderful influence of Professor Klumb had put me on an entirely new medical path. Ultimately, my undergraduate professors had challenged me not only to question established doctrine, but to develop new ways of thinking. They inspired me to be innovative and to explore all avenues of healing.

PROVING AUTOIMMUNITY

Upon completing my premedical studies in 1948, I entered medical school at the University of Freiberg. For the next several years, as I progressed with my studies, I became increasingly curious about the human immune system—that complex system of cells and cellular mechanisms that function to prevent chronic disease. I served as an intern at a large Hannover hospital for my last year of medical training. There, in 1952, I wrote my required doctoral thesis. The Director of the Pathology Department served as my thesis adviser. He was an extremely intuitive man who, prior to the War, had discovered that the mineral asbestos was a primary cause of lung cancer carcinogenesis (the production of cancer). Knowing of my interests in the human immune system, he assigned *Boeck's sarcoidosis* as my thesis topic. At the time, very little was known about this disease and its many manifestations.

I began research on this strange disease of unknown origin and postulated that it might be an *autoimmune disease*— that is, an illness caused by, or associated with, the development of an immune response to normal body tissues. Boeck's sarcoidosis is characterized by: chronic inflammation; the development of connective tissues with particularly large cells; and the growth of strangulating tissue that affects every organ from the heart to the joints. In extreme cases, Boeck's sarcoidosis can cause death by total tissue strangulation. (For more information on this disease, see

"Sarcoidosis," below.) I analyzed the pathology data on actual patients using advanced analytical techniques of the time. My important finding was that the body's immune system could actually consume and neutralize the parts of

Sarcoidosis

Sarcoidosis is a disorder of unknown origin, although it is thought that possibly a single agent or an immune deficiency may provoke this disease. It is also suspected that a genetic factor may be responsible. Sarcoidosis is characterized histologically by the presence of granulomas (tumors formed from granulation tissue) and small knotty nodules or tubercles, and involves various tissues and organs.

Depending on the site of the sarcoidosis and the degree of involvement, this disease can range from being asymptomatic to manifesting itself through serious, progressive multiorgan failure. Sarcoidosis can be acute or it can be chronic, occasionally going into remission. The lungs and thoracic lymph nodes are almost always involved when patients report acute respiratory problems accompanied by symptoms involving the skin, eyes, and other organs. Progress in immunology and molecular biology has increased our understanding of the pathology of this complex disease, as well as ways to diagnose and treat it.

The above information is gathered from my *Thesis on Boeck's Sarcoidosis* (written in 1952) and "Sarcoidosis," an article authored by L.S. Newman, C.S. Rose, and L.A. Maier and printed in the April 24, 1997 edition of *The New England Journal of Medicine*. For more information on these sources, see *Selected References*, page 163.

this system that normally protect the patient against tuberculosis.

At the time when I suggested that Boeck's sarcoidosis was an autoimmune disease, it was considered highly unlikely that any organism could consume itself—that an organism would actually attack itself as the host. People did not want to believe that the Lord would allow this to happen. Generally, the concept of autoimmunity was not accepted—even in medical circles—until ten to fifteen years later. So, in presenting my thesis, I took a chance of either being ridiculed for promoting such a radical view, or being recognized for my unprecedented conclusions.

My doctoral examination in 1952 was convened at the University of Hamburg, since there was no medical school in Hannover. I was successful in defending my thesis on Boeck's sarcoidosis as an autoimmune disease, and completed my doctoral examinations "summa cum laude," the highest award possible, before a panel of outstanding pathologists. This was the first time that an autoimmune disease had actually been proven to exist. My thesis was accepted for publication the following year in the very prestigious *Frankfurter Zeitzschrift fur Pathologie.*

My study of Boeck's sarcoidosis in medical school and my successful thesis defense of autoimmunity laid a firm foundation on which I would later build my research on actual mechanisms involved in immune system function. I was anxious to explore the role of cellular physics as it might pertain to the cellular transport of nutrients. I suspected that, through this approach, we could start finding ways to defend the body against cellular penetration by various disease-causing toxins, bacteria, and viruses. In retrospect, I now realize this was the beginning of my conviction that successful treatment of disease must be focused at the cellular level.

CHAPTER 3

*L*ESSONS FROM THE LAB

Truth in all its kinds is most difficult to win; and truth in medicine is the most difficult of all.

—Peter Mare Latham (1789–1875)

At twenty-four years of age, I had completed my formal medical training and was very anxious to continue my studies into the causes of autoimmune diseases. An appointment to the medical staff of the Hamelin City Hospital, Germany, enabled me to undertake basic clinical research on autoimmune diseases, which resulted in significant findings. I published these findings in a book on cell growth regulation. Also during this time, I became fascinated with the extensive accounts of the very challenging work being conducted in the relatively new field of *cancer chemotherapy*—the use of chemical agents and drugs selected to destroy cancer cells without seriously damaging normal cells.

CANCER RESEARCH APPOINTMENTS

I wanted to learn more about cancer chemotherapy and to actively participate in the exciting research. This eventually led me to seek appointments at a few of the leading cancer research institutions of that time. Through my various assignments, I was fortunate enough to work with some of the leading researchers in the cancer field and, together, we gained great knowledge about how cancer harms the body and how we can work to stop it.

Freiburg University Laboratory

In 1955, I had the opportunity to join the Cancer Research Team at Freiburg University Laboratory in Freiburg, Germany. Our research was conducted under the direction of Professor Hermann Druckrey, one of the most outstanding cancer researchers in postwar Germany. During the war, he had been Associate Professor of Pharmacology at the University of Berlin, served two years as a medical officer on the Russian front, and, in 1944, headed the major Pharmacological Institute in Vienna. For a short time after the war, Druckrey had been jailed for his involvement with the National Socialists. So as director of the hospital laboratories at Freiburg University, Professor Druckrey was trying to restore his reputation and reestablish himself as a leader in the field of cancer chemotherapy.

Our work was funded by the German Research Council. In Druckrey's laboratory, my colleagues and I conducted research on a number of new and potentially active anticancer agents. Among the substances were Cytoxan, nitrogen mustards, and a series of melamine compounds submitted for evaluation by Dr. Franz Kohler, Sr., a famous chemist who had synthesized the acrylates (Plexigas). Cytoxan showed limited promise in its effect on animal cancers. The nitrogen mustards were found to be strong toxic anticancer agents at Sloan-Kettering Institute in New

York. The melamines proved to be effective slow-acting anticancer agents, taking several weeks to have an effect. They were also considerably more difficult to control and produced toxic side effects. In addition, we were working with several nontoxic substances that exhibited great merit in testing, but they were swept under the carpet because they didn't meet the criteria of displaying rapid tumor inhibition within a few days after the start of testing. It would take these substances several months to have an effect.

Our team was about to publish the results on the melamines as promising but slow-acting chemotherapy agents with some toxic effects when Professor Druckrey intervened, asking that we suppress our research results. I was appalled that a man of his professional stature would even consider making such an unethical request. Only later, when I was no longer in Druckrey's laboratories, did I discover his apparent reason for doing this: Druckrey was seeking the Chair of the Pharmacology Department at the prestigious Heidelberg University, and he was fearful that our rather negative report on the melamines might jeopardize his chances of appointment. After all, everyone in the field at that time wanted to find the "magic bullet," the fast-acting cure with no toxic side effects. This experience foretold of future events that I would later witness, as I faced another coverup of significant research results for political and economic reasons. (See pages 39–41.) However, through my work on the melamines, I became closely acquainted with Dr. Franz Kohler, Sr., and began what would become a mutually beneficial, close working relationship that would last for many years to come.

Paul Ehrlich Institute of Experimental Therapy

In 1958, I joined the Paul Ehrlich Institute of Experimental Therapy in Frankfurt, Germany. I continued my research for two years there, exploring the function of the immune system and its inability to recognize the rapid growth and spread of cancer cells. During this same period, I became aware of the excellent clinical work being done at the nearby Asschaffenburg City Hospital. Later, in 1961, I would have the opportunity to conduct clinical research studies at Asschaffenburg, which would lead Dr. Kohler and I to develop important new therapeutic mineral carrier substances (calcium 2-aminoethylphosphate, in particular). But I spent my research time well at the Paul Ehrlich Institute. As I neared the completion of my work there in 1960, I became determined to seek an appointment at the prestigious Sloan-Kettering Institute in New York City.

Sloan-Kettering Institute for Cancer Research

In the 1960s, the Sloan-Kettering Institute for Cancer Research in New York City represented the ultimate opportunity for the young scientist interested in pursuing a career in cancer research. In fact, it was the leading cancer research center in the world at that time. I had good credentials and experience as a German physician of thirty-two years of age, but the competition for the few available visiting scientist appointments was fierce. I knew that I must seek help from some influential persons in the United States.

Several of the Jewish physicians who my father had helped escape from pre-war Nazi Germany in the 1930s were living in the New York area at that time. They came to my aid and were instrumental not only in helping me gain an appointment to the Sloan-Kettering Institute, but also in arranging all of my travel. In that moment, I thought of my father's kindness to his former colleagues, and their kindness in return. It struck me how life sometimes has a way of balancing out. How fortunate I was!

While at Sloan-Kettering Institute, in an extraordinary multidisciplinary research atmosphere, I consulted with a number of prominent cancer-research professionals. Our meetings continued throughout the 1970s. Among my colleagues was Dr. C. Chester Stock, who was Scientific Director of the Institute and an outstanding biochemist. He had been instrumental in designing and implementing the massive national chemotherapy screening program adopted by the National Cancer Institute (NCI) in its search for new, potentially active anticancer agents. I also worked with Lloyd Old, MD, who later became vice-president of the Sloan-Kettering Institute. Dr. Old worked with me on researching ways to stimulate the natural immune systems of experimental animals to fight against their cancers. Yet another brilliant colleague of mine was Dr. Kanematsu Sugiura, who is considered one of the great pioneering researchers in experimental chemotherapy.

At the time, I did not know that, some ten years later, I would be involved, again, with the Sloan-Kettering Institute and Dr. Sugiura. Together, we would fight what I shall call the *Apricot Pit War*, concerning the anticancer activity of a natural substance called *Laetrile*. This substance was first extracted from the apricot pit in the 1920s, by the late Dr. E.T. Krebs, Sr., of San Francisco. (See page 38.)

THE HISTORY OF CHEMOTHERAPY

Cancer chemotherapy arose shortly after World War II, when it was discovered that mustard gas—a poisonous gas used during World War I—disrupted cell growth. In 1948, a few of the leading scientific researchers from the Chemical Warfare Center in Frederick, Maryland, staffed the newly formed Sloan-Kettering Institute for Cancer Research in New York City. The research team soon reported finding a substance that was related to nitrogen mustard and displayed an inhibitory effect on several types of cancer, particularly leukemias and lymphomas.

The Approach

Because penicillin had so radically changed the face and thinking of medicine in the late 1940s, saving the lives of thousands of patients who would have died from over-whelming infections only a few years earlier, chemothera-py researchers adopted a similar strategy for the treatment and cure of cancer. They aimed namely to identify the offending cancer cells, to find new drugs ("magic bullets" that function like penicillin), and to use these drugs to kill the offending cells. But I learned in my research studies that cancer cells, unfortunately, are not alien invaders. They are normal cells that have undergone an abnormal transformation, and, as such, are not recognized by the body's immune system as foreign. Thus, the body permits their uncontrolled growth.

Cancer chemotherapy *antimetabolites* are normal cellular metabolic substances that have been chemically altered to render them cellular poisons. Based on the knowledge that cancer cells grow and multiply at many times the rate of normal cells, it was expected that cancer cells would rav-enously consume the majority of these carefully designed "poisonous" metabolites and be differentially destroyed. But while important differences between cancerous and normal cells do exist, there are even more similarities. As a result, the toxic chemotherapy agents (as well as radiation techniques) that aggressively target cancer cells always cause collateral damage to normal cells and to the body's immune system.

The Agents

I have evaluated many classes of chemotherapy agents over the past four decades. Most are either chemically syn-thesized in the laboratory, derived from natural substances such as plant extracts, or produced from cultured fungi or bacteria. For example, actinomycin D is a toxic antibiotic derived from certain soil bacteria. It is used to inhibit the cancer cell's genetic DNA and, hence, its cellular replication. Typical chemotherapy agents include: the chemical antimetabolites, which are substances that interfere with the cancer cell's life and reproductive cycles; the alkylating agents, which directly attack the cancer cell's DNA; naturally occurring plant alkaloids that block the cancer cell's mitotic division; inorganic chemical compounds; and specific steroidal hormones, which modify the growth of some hormone-dependent cancers.

All of these agents are generally quite toxic, and extreme care must be exercised in their use. I have experienced some success using limited chemotherapy with restraint, so as to not damage the immune system. It can shrink or slow the growth of certain cancers, particularly after surgery, but seldom does it offer a complete cure. In most cases, the disease outlasts the period of effective treatment. Thus, I came to the realization that aggressive cancer chemotherapy is not the answer.

A NEW PROMISE: LAETRILE (AMYGDALIN) AND THE MANDELONITRILES

From the 1920s to the 1940s, Dr. E.T. Krebs, Sr., and his son, Ernst Krebs, Jr., studied the cancer resistance of certain tribes and animal species. They found that the Hunza in Karakorum and the Eskimos are practically free of cancer in their native environments. Importantly, the Hunza tribe and the Eskimos, in distinction from all other people, absorb large quantities of *nitrilosides*—natural, biochemical, cyanide-containing substances found naturally in seeds (apricot kernels; nuts; bitter almonds), fodder, grasses, alfalfa, millet, etc. The Hunza draw these substances from apricot stones, while the Eskimos consume them in

certain arctic berries. It was found that *rhodanase*—an
enzyme present in high concentrations around cancer
cells—splits the nitrilosides into their components: hydro-
cyanic acid (HCN); benzaldehyde; and a sugar. The HCN
and benzaldehyde have anticancer qualities.

The Development of Laetrile and Related Substances

In the 1920s, Dr. Ernst Krebs, Sr., tested an oral extract of
apricot kernels. He found it to be quite toxic, but effective
against malignancies. Ernst Krebs, Jr., developed a less
toxic extract, which he called *Laetrile* (short for Laevomandelonitrile). Laetrile—also termed vitamin B_{17}; amygdalin;
and l-glucose mandelonitrile—consists of a single glucose
molecule chemically bonded to a molecule of HCN and
benzaldehyde, just like the nitrilosides in the Hunza's apricot stones and the Eskimos' arctic berries. The toxic HCN
is released only when the compound is split by the rhodanase enzyme present at cancer cell locations, thus selec-
tively destroying the cancer cells. The benzaldehyde, a
powerful pain killer and nontoxic anticancer substance, is
also released primarily at the cancer cell site.

During the 1960s, the Drs. Cassetti of Florence, Italy, discovered that the l-glucose mandelonitrile (that is, Laetrile)
is metabolized only by cancer cells and not by normal cells,
thus explaining its unique anticancer properties. In the late
1960s, I clinically evaluated Laetrile and found it quite
effective in the treatment of various types of human cancer.
Because it was difficult for me to obtain Laetrile from the
United States at that time, I asked the late Dr. Franz Kohler,
Sr., my friend and collaborator from my laboratory days at
Freiburg University, Germany, to design a mandelonitrile
molecule in which the l-glucose portion of the structure
was replaced by urea. He successfully synthesized a series
of mandelonitriles of varying chemical compositions,

based on the original l-glucose (Laetrile) structure, in the hope of producing more highly effective, nontoxic anticancer agents.

From among the series, I submitted ureyl-, nicotinyl-, and para-aminobenzoic-mandelonitriles to Sloan-Kettering Institute for thorough experimental evaluation as potential nontoxic anticancer agents. They showed such great promise that I subsequently used a mixture of the ureyl- and nicotinyl-mandelonitriles in place of Laetrile in my clinical practice. All of these synthetic mandelonitriles are very effective aldehyde donors, which also makes them very effective gene-repair substances. (See Chapter 7.)

Success and Controversy

By the early 1970s, Laetrile proponents were promoting the substance as a promising nontoxic anticancer agent. However, the substance became the focus of a national controversy in the United States. During the testing of this substance, the venerable Dr. Sugiura discovered that it prevented lung metastases in a line of genetically related mice who had developed spontaneous mammary tumors and had exhibited a high incidence of lung cancer metastases. Strangely, the Sloan-Kettering Institute pressured him to suppress his report.

For some time, the American Cancer Society, the National Cancer Institute, the American Medical Society, and several state medical societies had conducted a widespread campaign against Laetrile, claiming that this nontoxic substance was without merit and that its use constituted "cancer quackery." Sloan-Kettering's actions may have been part of a coordinated attack launched because Laetrile offered little or no economic return to the pharmaceutical companies. The powerful Food and Drug Administration (FDA) claimed it "had seen no competent, scientific evidence of Laetrile's effectiveness against cancer" and banned the substance. The California Public Health Department's report similarly concluded that "Laetriles are of no value in the diagnosis, treatment, alleviation or cure of cancer."

In 1974, Dr. Dean Burk, Head of the Cytochemistry Branch of the National Cancer Institute (NCI), produced strong evidence of the effectiveness of Laetrile as an anticancer agent. He spoke out strongly in support of its efficacy and against the apparent coverup. Later that year, over 40,000 signatures were gathered nationwide in petitions to then President Richard Nixon and his wife. The petitions urged for a lifting of the ban on Laetrile. The controversy became a major political issue.

California doctors using Laetrile in defiance of the ban were arrested, their medical licenses were revoked, and their patient records and medical supplies were confiscated. As the Federal and State governments prosecuted these doctors for the use of alternative, "unproven" therapies, Laetrile was being used legally in neighboring Mexico and several other Western countries. In their zeal to "protect" Americans, the FDA and the ICC (Interstate Commerce Commission) completely prohibited all interstate commerce in Laetrile. Tragically, U.S. citizens who purchased Laetrile in Mexico and brought it back home were arrested on their return to the United States for bringing the "illegal" drug across the border. "Freedom of choice" became the hew and cry across America. The primary question was, "Does a terminally ill cancer patient have the right to access a therapeutic substance exhibiting no side effects in the treatment of his or her own cancer?"

Meanwhile, at Sloan-Kettering Institute, when the order was issued to suppress Dr. Sugiura's positive test results on Laetrile, a leading Institute spokesman, Dr. Ralph Moss, PhD, bluntly revealed this coverup and left the Sloan-Kettering Institute not of his own accord. Moss went on to author several works on the industry of cancer treatments. I have been profoundly moved by Ralph Moss' book entitled

Questioning Chemotherapy. His detailed knowledge, immense expertise in the field, and great integrity qualify him to describe the sweeping failure of orthodox "toximolecular" medicine in treating chronic diseases. I, too, have frequently observed the disastrous effects of toxic chemotherapy on many of my patients from the United States who, as a last resort, have traveled to my clinic in Germany, seeking alternative treatment for their cancers and other life-threatening chronic diseases.

Support for the Mandelonitriles

My former colleague Dr. C. Chester Stock has retired from Sloan-Kettering in recent years. Since then, he and I have corresponded about the Laetrile affair. I have shared with him the great success I've experienced in using the mandelonitriles, particularly the ureyl-mandelonitrile, in my clinical practice. Ureyl-mandelonitrile has been my most effective agent in treating prostate and pancreatic cancers, Hodgkin's disease, and chronic leukemias. When treated with ureyl-mandelonitrile, these diseases respond well and remain in stable remission as never seen before. It all began with Laetrile.

I think back to 1973, when Alecia Buttons, wife of comedian Red Buttons, came to me for treatment of her cancer. Later, she stated that the mandelonitriles that she was given had saved her life. She is alive and well today. And this is only one of many examples. There was great support for Laetrile from the beginning; if only the U.S. government organizations had listened and had kept an open mind. Disturbingly, throughout the 1970s, more than 365,000 Americans died of cancer each year. Consider the fact that, at the same time that Laetrile (amygdalin) was banned by the FDA and could not be used to help these people, governmental organizations made no effort to curtail smoking, which is known to be a primary cause of lung cancer. The statistics are alarming: in 1960, over 36,000 Americans died of lung cancer; in 1990, over 140,000 died of lung cancer. That's almost a 400-percent increase in thirty years! Yet the tobacco industry booms, while alternative, natural, nontoxic cancer treatments are stifled.

For over ten years, Dr. Massimo Bonucci, a pathologist and surgeon from Pisa, Italy, has come to Hannover for two days each month, to work with me in the hospital and in my office. Over these years, I have seen him develop into a brilliant oncologist. In the spring of 1995, Bonucci brought a series of X-rays documenting the dramatic regression and then the complete remission of a vast adenocarcinoma—a metastatic cancer of the lung involving cancerous growth of glandular tissue—on the upper-right pulmonary lobe of one of his patients. Bonucci explained that orthodox chemotherapy had not only failed, but it had apparently resulted in an enhancement of the disease. The patient was next given a number of substances: thymus, a glandular extract; squalene, which is shark liver oil; ascorbate, more commonly known as vitamin C; didrovaltrate, an herbal extract containing bifunctional aldehydes; and a small amount of Carnivora, a Venus fly-trap plant extract containing cell-blocking, anticancer enzymes. These treatments produced some improvement, but not enough to explain the amazing X-ray results. Dr. Bonucci then revealed that he had given his patient ureyl-mandelonitrile at three times the normal dose level and at a much increased frequency than I normally recommended. The complete remission of the disease took only ten short weeks. This experience serves as a fine example of the promise of nontoxic orthomolecular cancer treatments.

THE FUTURE OF MEDICINE

The whole Laetrile affair is not without some positive irony; today's research gives high priority to *gene-repairing* agents in treating cancer, and deals primarily with the *functional aldehydes* (see page 101), of which Laetrile— damned by U.S. orthodox medicine—was among the first. For over twenty years, ureyl-mandelonitrile has been the mainstay at my clinic at Hannover and for my work at the Paracelsus Silbersee Hospital. I continue to observe the greatest clinical results I have seen in forty years when higher doses are administered more frequently.

In my numerous published writings, I have occasionally predicted that the downfall of the orthodox school of cancer treatment would be precipitated not so much by its failure to cure, but simply by its exorbitant costs. The tremendous explosion of healthcare costs threatens to destroy healthcare programs and even national economies worldwide. This problem is the direct result of a rigid commitment to costly orthodox therapies that simply don't work and, furthermore, have little or no usefulness as preventive therapies. It is not unusual to encounter enormous bills for the toxic conventional treatment of breast cancer: $200,000 to $400,000 in New York, New York and Boston, Massachusetts; and 325,000 DM in Heidelburg, Germany. Consider, too, the exorbitant cost of treating ovarian cancer: $84,000 in Orlando, Florida. These costs hurt both us and our nations. And my opinion is that the rate of improvement following these conventional treatments is minimal, the suffering of patients under toxic chemotherapy is often severe, and the overall quality of life is deplorable. If it can be seen that a ship is about to sink, as is the case with toxic chemotherapy, then some thought should be given to finding a lifeboat. The latter can be found in nontoxic therapeutic procedures and orthomolecular therapies that repair the genetic misinformation contained in the genes of the cancerous cells. Orthomolecular approaches work to restore proper balance to the body's chemistry, thus restoring health.

Through my years of research and clinical practice, I have learned how to best protect the body against life-threatening cellular deterioration. Furthermore, I have learned how to treat and heal my patients using a broad spectrum of nontoxic, orthomolecular, metabolic substances, including gene-repairing substances and *mineral transporters,* discussed in detail in Chapter 5. The following chapters will explain some of these exciting discoveries and will help you in sharing my vision of a much brighter future that promotes the successful prevention and treatment of life-threatening diseases.

NUTRIENT METABOLISM AND TRANSPORT

. . . genuine understanding of disease mechanisms is relatively inexpensive, relativity simple, and relatively easy to deliver.

from *The Lives of a Cell*
—Dr. Lewis Thomas (1913–1993)

It is important for me to share my research findings so that you can make more informed decisions concerning the prevention and treatment of several chronic diseases. But in order to understand some of the scientific breakthroughs that I have achieved in developing new therapeutic substances in my laboratories, first it is necessary to learn how our bodies carry out the basic daily functions that sustain life. This chapter details how the body breaks down nutrients and transport them into the cells.

THE BREAKDOWN OF NUTRIENTS

Most of the nutrients and all of the energy that the body needs to carry out its many complex functions are provided by the foods and liquids we routinely consume. The digestive system is quite marvelous in the way it breaks down these foods and liquids into smaller and smaller molecular components. The components are absorbed into the bloodstream for distribution to the cells throughout the body.

Metabolism involves physical and chemical processes through which substances are either broken down and converted into energy or combined with other components for essential use. The minute nutrient molecules must be in a form that our cells can utilize. Thus, substances called *digestive enzymes* break down fats, carbohydrates, and proteins into ions that carry positive or negative electrical charges. For example, pepsin and trypsin, both pancreatic enzymes, break down proteins into smaller molecules called peptides and polypeptides; amylase, another pancreatic enzyme, breaks down starches into maltose, a disaccharide sugar; lipase, still another pancreatic enzyme, breaks down fats into fatty acids and glycerol; and finally, hydrochloric acid, together with pepsin, kills unwanted bacteria. Quite differently, most salts and mineral nutrients form ions or electrolytes that are absorbed directly into our blood serum and circulate throughout our bodies. In these cases, enzymes are not necessary.

We frequently hear about the importance of maintaining a proper electrolyte balance, which is linked to a healthy metabolism. *Electrolytes* are liquid solutions of ions that are able to conduct electricity. They are similar to the acid solution in a car's battery which, together with the lead battery plates, creates the electricity required to operate the car's engine. Diseases and nutritional deficiencies often cause blood electrolyte imbalances.

In my clinical research and practice, I have found that certain mineral and nutrient supplements are essential in protecting the body from the degenerative effects of disease and aging. For these supplements to be effective, they must be designed to seek out and, by directed transport, to carry their minerals to specific organs, cells, and the cells' functional components. I consider nutrient and mineral transporters to be among my most potent weapons in the prevention and treatment of disease.

MINERAL TRANSPORT

Let me give you a tour of the principles that govern how *active directed mineral transport* works and what it can do. These principles were introduced in the late 1950s by Dr. Laborit of Paris, Dr. Blumberger of Hannover, and myself. They have been extended progressively to all branches of medicine and to almost all disease states.

The Basics on Disease and Mineral Transporters

According to Dr. Hans Selye of Montreal, a disease may be described and explained by a small number of fundamental pathological disturbances of the cell—for example, a change in cellular membrane permeability; a change in structure; a cancerous process; or any other significant change in metabolic function. It follows that there are specific transport agents that can improve or cure the disease at the cellular level. This principle can apply to the treatment of most diseases. In fact, it is the basis of today's advanced orthomolecular medicine, which holds that disease may be cured by restoring to the body an optimum balance of those essential substances required to maintain its normal functions.

A mineral transport substance works by releasing an ion—an atom or group of atoms that carries a positive or negative charge—at a particular cell site where the ion is required. It is figuratively possible, by design, to write an address on the mineral ion and have it directed to where it will carry out specific functions, such as: activating biological enzymes; restoring damaged cell structure; conducting genetic repair; or sealing cellular membranes against potential harm by toxins, bacteria, or viruses. Mineral transport has a very simple principle and is extremely harmless, while producing extraordinary results.

The actual *process* of the transportation and absorption of essential minerals involves complex biochemical systems existing within all of the body's cells. In order to gain a better understanding of the role of mineral transporters in preventive medicine, it is necessary to explain the fundamentals of the human cell.

The Structure and Function of the Cell

Most human cells are composed of many small functional elements surrounded by a complex, double-layered membrane. The primary functional elements within the cell include: the mitochondria (or mitocondrial organelles), the cell's "furnaces," which break down sugars and fats to produce cellular energy, termed ATP (adenosine triphosphate); the lysosomes (or lysosome organelles), which produce important enzymes that break down and destroy bacteria and other unwanted substances; the endoplasmic reticulum, which helps transport nutrients and other materials inside the cell; the ribosomes, which are essential in binding proteins together; the vacuoles, which store and transport water into and excrete wastes out of the interior of the cell; the vesicles (or vesicle sacs) on the exterior of the cell membrane, which contain enzymes that function to excrete wastes at the membrane surface; the chromosomes, which contain the genetic DNA and RNA of the cells and are contained within the cell's nucleus; the centrioles, which are sets of hollow tubules essential to cellular (mitotic) division; and, lastly, the all-important nucleus, which serves as the cell's central control system. (See Figure 4.1.)

The cell membrane is the gatekeeper of the cell. As illustrated in Figure 4.2 (see page 50), it consists of an outer and

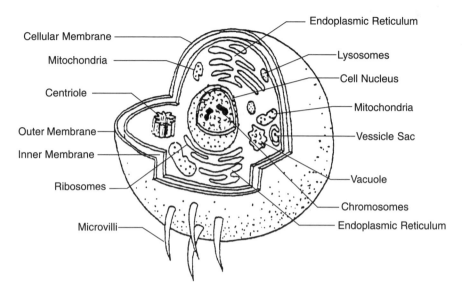

Figure 4.1. Typical Cell Structure

an inner layer of phospholipids, which form a gel-like substance. Hydrophobic (water-rejecting) fatty-acid molecular chains exist in the space between the inner and outer membrane layers. Glycoprotein carbohydrate chains attach to the external surface. The membranes of all cells retain an electrical field with a strength of about one-tenth of a volt. This electrical charge serves to regulate the transport of substances that are essential for healthy cell growth and replication, the excretion of wastes from the cell, and the prevention and treatment of diseases at the cellular level. For more information, see "Cell Membranes—The Gatekeepers," page 51.)

The Actual Transport of Nutrients

As mentioned at the beginning of this chapter, nutrients are useful only when they can be incorporated at the cellular level. Thus, they must enter the interior of the cell. There are three types of membrane transport. The first is

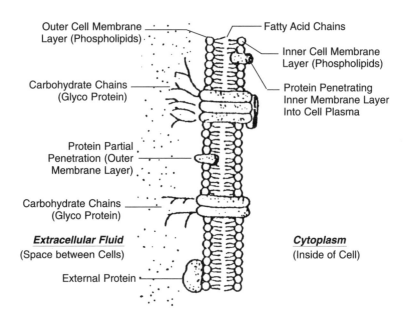

Outer Cell Membrane Layer (Phospholipids)

Fatty Acid Chains

Inner Cell Membrane Layer (Phospholipids)

Carbohydrate Chains (Glyco Protein)

Protein Penetrating Inner Membrane Layer Into Cell Plasma

Protein Partial Penetration (Outer Membrane Layer)

Carbohydrate Chains (Glyco Protein)

Extracellular Fluid (Space between Cells)

Cytoplasm (Inside of Cell)

External Protein

Figure 4.2. Typical Cell Membrane Structure

passive diffusion, which permits fat-soluble substances to diffuse through the bi-layered phospholipid membrane of the cell without a transport carrier. Next, there is *facilitated diffusion*, which requires a special transport substance to serve as a carrier of water-soluble substances. Third and finally, there is *active transport*, which requires the input of cellular energy (ATP) to accomplish the transport of certain substances.

Positively charged mineral ions, such as calcium, magnesium, and potassium, may have considerable difficulty in passing through the positively charged surface of cellular membranes which, like the positive poles of ordinary magnets, repel the like-charged mineral ions. To overcome this, I began to search for new classes of mineral supplements consisting of negatively charged *carrier ions* bound to positively charged *mineral ions*. Such supplements could be transported as electrically-neutral (nonpolar) substances by simple diffusion through the cellular membrane.

Cell Membranes— The Gatekeepers

The average human body contains some 3,000 square meters of membranes—cellular equivalents of "electrical fences"—that maintain the borders of the cells and the organs they form. Without the framework of these membranes, we would be nothing more than very large, very disorganized puddles. Moreover, in addition to their structural importance, membranes play a critical role as gatekeepers of the cells. By maintaining a very precise electrical balance, these amazing structures control both the intra- and extracellular environments, permitting certain nutrients to enter, shunting waste products out, and communicating with the other cells of the body.

The details of the structure and function of cell membranes were not fully understood until the development of the electron microscope, which allowed scientists to observe the cell membrane and its composition. What they found was an astonishingly complex, bi-layered structure of carefully arrayed lipids, carbohydrates, and proteins. Few molecules can pass easily through this barrier. Most require the assistance of protein transporters, which shuttle molecules back and forth across the membrane or through the openings of protein pores called *ion channels*. These channels open in response to chemical signals or to changes in the membrane's electrical charge.

Ion channels that open in response to electrical charges are known as *voltage-dependent channels*. These are the cell's universal translators that accept, translate, and pass the signals from the extracellular world, including the all-important electrical signals of the nervous system. They are controlled by a handful of minerals known as electrolytes: sodium, potassium, calcium, and magnesium, which are positively charged; and chloride, phosphate, and amino acids, which are negatively charged.

Sodium- and potassium-controlled channels work together to maintain the cell membrane's electrical charge (or membrane potential) at an average of 90 kilovolts per centimeter. Calcium channels open in response to changes in membrane potential, allowing calcium into the cell, where it is involved in a host of cellular reactions. Healthy cellular function depends on the proper balance of these minerals, both inside and outside the cell.

The importance of maintaining proper membrane potential may best be understood by considering the consequences of its disruption, which can range from muscular weakness and spasms to complete failure of the heart muscle. Many neurological disorders, such as Parkinson's disease, multiple sclerosis, and epilepsy, are actually due to disruptions of cellular communication in which nerve cells are sending or receiving inappropriate electrical messages.

Substances That Affect Transport

As early as 1955, Dr. Hans Selye (mentioned previously) and Dr. S. von Nida of Munich demonstrated that magnesium chloride could protect the hearts of experimental animals from chemically induced necrosis, or tissue degeneration. Guided by their work, I developed an *active mineral transport system* to restore magnesium to heart and circulatory cells, utilizing two excellent organic carrier molecules

—phenylalanine and paraminobenzoic acid. But I didn't stop there; I continued my search for other carriers that could provide more effective transport of magnesium and potassium to the cells of the heart. By 1958, I had succeeded in developing *potassium-magnesium aspartate* as an active mineral transport system. At the same time, in Paris, a colleague and brilliant researcher, Dr. Henri Laborit, developed the same active transport molecule, and patents were granted to each of us. I initially licensed Farbwerke Hoecht in Germany to produce the new potassium-magnesium aspartate, while Dr. Laborit licensed the Wyeth Laboratories in the United States.

Potassium-magnesium aspartate became known worldwide as a successful mineral substance for protecting against cardiac-tissue destruction and arrest. It was also found to improve liver function and to detoxify digitalis, a strong cardiac stimulant and diuretic prescribed to many heart patients. As the next chapter will tell, my work with potassium-magnesium aspartate was the first step in developing a series of highly effective mineral transporters that work to combat chronic disease.

CHAPTER 5

𝒯HE MINERAL TRANSPORTERS

Only orthomolecular substances can bring success in
long-term therapy . . . only these can achieve a true cure
in treating the ravaging effects of degenerative diseases . . . .

—Nobel Laureate Dr. Linus Pauling (1901–1994)

Continuing my work on active mineral transporters, I conceived of a broad spectrum of mineral substances similar to potassium-magnesium aspartate (discussed in Chapter 4), changing the various minerals to be transported and selecting new carrier molecules. The direct transport to very specific cell sites allowed minerals to be effectively incorporated and utilized by the targeted cells.

My colleague the late Dr. Franz Kohler, who had been so successful in preparing the mandelonitriles for me in the 1960s, was even more brilliant in his synthesis of the calcium, potassium, magnesium, zinc, and lithium mineral salts of *aspartic* and *orotic acids, arginine* (a basic amino acid), and *2-aminoethylphosphate* (2-AEP). In my opinion, these are the most important mineral transporters available today. This chapter briefly discusses the role of each of these mineral salts in the prevention and treatment of specific diseases at the cellular level. The information comes from the clinical observations and experiences that my Hannover staff and I have accumulated.

THE ASPARTATES

The aspartates are the mineral salts of aspartic acid. The active mineral transporter—the negative ion of aspartic acid—delivers its associated mineral to the inner portion of the double-walled cellular membrane.

Calcium-*l,dl*-Aspartate

I have found that calcium aspartate, above all other mineral aspartates, provides a pronounced effect in the control of and relief from painful fibrocystic calcification of the breast. I observed this beneficial effect in over 98 percent of my female patients who took calcium aspartate. Also, in the early 1960s, I noted that calcium aspartate was effective in the *recalcification* of bone tissue in the aftermath of bone tuberculosis. We use it today in the treatment of osteoporosis and osteomyelitis, with similar positive results.

Potassium-Magnesium Aspartate

Through potassium-magnesium aspartate, potassium and magnesium mineral ions are transported to the inner portion of the cells of the heart, arteries, and the liver. At these locations, they activate specific enzymes, which, in turn, produce energy-rich adenosinetriphosphate (ATP), essential in providing increased energy and oxygen to the blood. This action within the heart muscle becomes paramount in overcoming the risk of cardiac necrosis (destruction of heart tissue), coronary thrombosis (intravascular formation of a clot), arteriosclerosis (thickening of the arteries); and sudden cardiac arrest.

In addition, potassium-magnesium aspartate promotes the detoxification of the liver by removing ammonia, thus helping in the prevention of liver failure. Furthermore, by reducing tension in the lungs through the conversion of carbon dioxide into urea, which is then excreted, potassium-magnesium aspartate has been shown to help individuals in overcoming asthmatic attacks. So this substance greatly contributes to better health in a number of significant ways.

Zinc Aspartate

I have found zinc aspartate, in combination with magnesium orotate, to be extremely useful in the treatment of the small, non-Hodgkin's lymphomas (Burkitt's lymphomas) caused by the Epstein-Barr and cytomegalo viruses. Zinc aspartate and magnesium orotate are very effective in arresting the replication of viruses and also in inhibiting the activity of the enzyme thymadine kinase, which may explain their ability to combat the lymphomas. Following the surgical removal of a lymphoma, the immunological complement C3c in the patient's blood serum must be maintained above a minimum threshold level to avoid tumor recurrence. Together, zinc aspartate and magnesium orotate are very effective in accomplishing this.

In Germany, zinc aspartate is accepted and routinely offered as a mineral substance for the enhancement of the immune defense system. It activates the thymus gland and the formation of T-lymphocytes, which are important elements of the immune system. Finally, zinc aspartate seems to increase the body's production of insulin, which makes a valuable contribution to the treatment of diabetes.

THE OROTATES

During our preliminary work on electrolyte carriers based
on aspartic acid, Dr. Franz Kohler and I considered the
possibility that orotic acid might be an appropriate carrier
molecule. It was already known that orotic acid penetrates
very easily into the cell and, as an aromatic substance,
its salts possess high chemical-complexing power. We
found that the orotates pass through the cell's double-
layered outer membrane and are decomposed for utiliza-
tion only by the inner components of the cell, such as the
mitochondria.

Calcium Orotate

After years of clinical use, I conclude that calcium orotate
has proven to be one of three mineral transporters that are
the most active in providing treatment for bone decalcification. The other two are calcium aspartate and calcium 2-
aminoethylphosphate, or calcium 2-AEP. These three substances are far superior to conventional calcium salts and
anabolic hormones, and clinically exhibit far less side effects. Calcium orotate, and calcium 2-AEP moreso, are
most effective in recalcifying bone tissue following extensive radiation treatment of cancerous bone lesions. Through
electron microscopic inspection, we now know that only
calcium orotate penetrates directly through the cell membrane, delivering calcium to the interior of the cell where it
is readily utilized.

I have also found calcium orotate valuable for its pronounced anti-inflammatory effect on a number of disorders, including: arthritis; arteriosclerosis; retinitis, or inflammation of the retina; disseminated encephalitis, or
inflammation of the brain; and phlebitis, or inflammation
of a vein. In addition, it is very effective against psoriasis, a scaling skin disorder. The long-term clinical tolerance and overall value of calcium orotate is far superior

to other therapeutic calcium substances and to the so-called immune depressors.

Lithium Orotate

Since its initial introduction in my clinic, lithium orotate has played a major role in the treatment of depression. It does not trigger the harmful side effects that normally occur with high doses of lithium acetate, carbonate, or citrate, also used for depression. In addition, I have found lithium orotate particularly beneficial in the treatment of migraine and frequently recurring headaches.

Magnesium Orotate

Dr. Franz Kohler and I found that magnesium orotate reduces serum cholesterol levels more efficiently than any other substance we had used previously. This marked effect was observed even when this orotate was administered at relatively small dose levels of 200 to 600 mg per day. Magnesium orotate prevents hardening of the arteries, restoring the cells of the arteries even more successfully than calcium aspartate. We also found that magnesium orotate prevents kidney failure from chronic hypertension (high blood pressure) and diabetes. Finally, in combination with zinc aspartate, this substance helps stop the replication of viruses. (See page 57.)

Potassium Orotate

Through tests done on hamsters, Dr. Kohler and I demonstrated that potassium orotate, like potassium aspartate, could prevent spontaneous heart-tissue destruction. It has since been used extensively both as a preventative agent of heart muscle degradation and as the most effective potassium transporter to cell plasma. Ninety percent of the potassium found in the human body is inside the cells.

Potassium orotate penetrates the cell membrane and delivers required potassium to the cell, where it is utilized to maintain the fluid (plasma) pressure.

THE ARGINATES

From 1961 to 1962, Dr. Kohler and I developed the mineral salts of arginine, an alkaline amino acid. At first, we suspected that arginine might not form a salt. However, due to its complexing properties, we eventually succeeded in forming its potassium, magnesium, calcium, and zinc salts. These mineral substances proved highly beneficial in the treatment of a number of health problems.

Calcium Arginate

In very developed countries, we have found the glucose transport system in type II (late onset) diabetic patients to be defective. It is strongly suspected that this condition is due, in large part, to the ingestion of detergents over a period of years. (See page 75 for a discussion on the effect of detergents on health.) Many diabetics are able to control their blood sugar levels by following a specific diet and/or by taking insulin. But in severe cases, these treatment approaches are not enough. The normal glucose absorption mechanism is so resistant to insulin that the blood glucose levels climb dangerously high. Yet there is good news for those who suffer from this advanced problem. My colleagues and I have done clinical studies, which were published in Germany's *Raum und Zeit* and scheduled for publication in the *Townsend Letter for Doctors* as well, that have shown that calcium arginate, as well as magnesium arginate and zinc arginate, lower the blood glucose levels of those with such cases of diabetes.

Since arginine is a normal component and plays an important role in the glucose transport mechanism, arginates can easily serve as acceptors for glucose. So I have given diabetic patients both calcium arginate and magnesium arginate, with spectacular results thus far. Blood glucose levels fall dramatically, without any apparent side effects. I expect long-term observations will confirm this therapeutic breakthrough. It is particularly pleasing to have found a simple, inexpensive, nutrient-based therapy for type II diabetes.

Furthermore, several patients from both the United States and Germany have written me claiming that calcium arginate has provided significant improvement regarding inner-ear hearing loss. To verify these claims, clinical studies have been instituted and are in progress at several university otological departments in Germany, including those at Hannover's HNO Hospital and MHH Hospital. This is an exciting additional area of study.

Magnesium Arginate

As discussed previously, magnesium arginate plays a significant role in lowering blood glucose levels, thus providing better management of diabetes. Please see the "Calcium Arginate" section for further detail. Also, I have found that magnesium arginate definitely enhances the effectiveness of *l-carnitine,* an essential vitamin that transports fatty acids into the mitochondria of the cells, enabling the body to utilize fats for energy. This is particularly important for the functioning of the heart muscle, which derives its energy primarily from fatty acids. For this reason, many people now take arginates to enhance heart health. (For more information, see the December 1997 issue of the *Townsend Letter for Doctors,* page 46.)

Zinc Arginate

Zinc arginate has been found to be very effective in lowering blood glucose levels. This allows for safe, natural, and effective treatment of diabetes. Please see the "Calcium Arginate" section for details on arginate applications for diabetes.

2-AMINOETHYLPHOSPHATE (2-AEP, OR COLAMINE PHOSPHATE)

In 1939, famous biochemist Dr. Erwin Chargoff reported that aminoethylphosphate (AEP) is an essential component in the structure of all cell membranes. Further studies were conducted by Swiss scientist Dr. Buchi in 1952, and they yielded further information about the chemical and functional structure of cellular membranes and the role of aminoethylphosphate. I was thus convinced of the advantages to developing active mineral transporters from this substance.

Calcium 2-Aminoethylphosphate (Calcium 2-AEP)

Impressed with the findings of Chargoff and Buchi, I asked my colleague Dr. Franz Kohler to prepare the calcium salt of 2-aminoethylphosphate for clinical trial. He was successful in the synthesis of calcium 2-AEP—one of the most important and effective mineral transport substances I have ever conceived. As with any new clinical substance, I had to determine its functional characteristics. I was able to demonstrate that calcium 2-AEP, serving as an electrolyte carrier and mineral transporter, decreases cellular membrane permeability by sealing the membrane's free-lipid pore sites. Free-lipid pores are defective pores that permit harmful agents to penetrate the cell membrane and produce disease. Therefore, calcium 2-AEP prevents disease-causing bacteria, toxins, and viruses from penetrating the cell. In 1967 and 1968, I published information on this substance in the Parisian journal titled *Agressologie* (see Selected References, page 167).

At Muenster, Germany, in 1972, Dr. Moenninghoff provided extensive electron microscopic evidence confirming how the cell membrane's free-lipid pore sites could be successfully sealed with calcium 2-AEP. Then, from later communications with Dr. Pressman (in New York), we learned that the mineral phosphates, including calcium, magnesium, and potassium 2-AEPs, are components of our neurotransmitters—substances necessary for the conduction of the nerves' electrical signals. Calcium 2-AEP is particularly necessary to retain the electrical charge on the membrane surface. The mineral phosphates are indispensable in supporting the condenser function of cells at the membrane surface.

My first clinical application of calcium 2-AEP took place in 1964. It aimed at the treatment of multiple sclerosis (MS). In the past thirty-five years, I have treated more than 3,150 MS patients, over 68 percent of whom are from North America. Basically, results have been far better than those of any other MS therapy employed. (See pages 124 to 125 for an explanation of the conventional approaches used to treat this disease.) Among MS patients treated conventionally, about 25 percent die of bone fractures, and another 25 percent die of kidney failure. Amazingly, I have seen only eight cases of bone fractures and no situations of kidney failure in my patients on calcium 2-AEP.

Years later, in 1986, Dr. George Morrisette of the United States conducted a retrospective study of 300 MS patients who had begun their calcium 2-AEP therapy in my Hannover clinic. His study showed that 82 percent had positive benefits from this therapy, and in patients who had begun this therapy shortly after diagnosis, the results rose to 92 percent. Since multiple sclerosis is so prevalent in the United States, particularly in the dairy-belt states, and because the orthodox school of medicine has been unable to offer promising prevention or treatment for this debilitating chronic disease, I devote Chapter 8 to a thorough discussion of my findings and therapies used in the treatment of MS.

Multiple sclerosis is only one of several chronic disorders that can be prevented or treated with calcium 2-AEP therapy. Let's consider osteoporosis and the loss of calcium in the bones. Over 1.3 million spontaneous bone fractures due to osteoporosis and decalcification of the bone, mostly in the elderly, are reported annually in the United States. Both men and women experience a loss in bone density during middle age. However, post-menopausal women are particularly vulnerable to osteoporosis and bone decalcification, due to a decline in estrogen production. To combat these problems, many women are given estrogen. But such hormonal therapy has exhibited only minimal enhancement of calcium retention, and is not entirely free from negative side effects. I have found calcium 2-AEP, together with calcium orotate, to be the therapy of choice in the prevention and treatment of osteoporosis and related decalcification diseases.

How does it work? Calcium 2-AEP improves the condenser function of the bone-cell membranes, allowing the bone cells to function healthily. Thus, this therapy dramatically reduces the risk of bone fractures. Furthermore, surgeons in six major medical centers—two in the United States, in the cities of St. Louis and Tampa—reported finding extremely solid bone when implanting new joints in patients who had been taking calcium 2-AEP and calcium orotate for at least four years prior to their surgeries. So calcium 2-AEP increases bone *density* as well. I have seen this evidenced through elderly osteoporosis patients who have taken this treatment.

Diabetes is yet another disease that can be prevented or treated with the calcium 2-AEP therapy, whether used individually or as part of a highly effective complex. During the late 1960s, I noticed that patients with rather severe diabetes felt better when treated with calcium 2-AEP.

Their overall metabolism improved, tolerance to sugar increased, and their kidneys appeared to react favorably to this treatment.

The actual problem in diabetes, which is so common today, is not so much the increased blood sugar, but the systemic consequences resulting from it. Excessive glucose levels produce unacceptable sugar deposits in numerous structures of the body, ranging from the red blood hemoglobin to the cell membranes of the blood vessel systems. This results in the degeneration of the small vessels, turning diabetes into a severe, drawn-out illness that may not become evident for twenty years or so.

The damage to the blood vessel and capillary systems due to diabetes can easily be observed in the small vessels of the eye's retina. In the United States, diabetes is the second most frequent cause of blindness. The condition is called *diabetic retinopathy*. Furthermore, the function of the brain, particularly concerning intellectual ability, can be seriously impaired by such diabetic damage to the small vessels, as well as to the large carotid artery, which feeds the brain with oxygen-rich blood. I found that calcium 2-AEP, in combination with magnesium 2-AEP and potassium 2-AEP to form a three-part complex, is highly effective in combating this diabetic progression. The following section on the 2-AEP complex will further explain these findings. It is also important to note that Dr. Robert Atkins, in New York, has demonstrated that calcium 2-AEP, specifically, significantly reverses juvenile diabetes type I. My staff and I have made similar observations.

2-AEP Complex: Calcium, Magnesium, Potassium 2-AEP (Ca, Mg, K 2-AEP)

Having collaborated for many years with several ophthalmologists in Germany and the United States, I am certain that the calcium, magnesium, potassium 2-AEP therapy is extremely effective in preserving the retina by restoring retinal cell membrane integrity. The prevention of diabetic retinopathy solely with Ca, Mg, K 2-AEP has given me and my collaborators great satisfaction. This is why I have called this complex the Membrane Integrity (M_i) factor.

The kidneys are also protected by the administration of the mineral 2-AEP complex, in combination with magnesium orotate, in both diabetic and heart patients. The 2-AEP complex can decrease high blood pressure and eliminate excess protein in the urine of diabetic patients with initial kidney damage.

The mineral 2-AEP complex also improves the regulation of blood glucose in the treatment of type II diabetes. For elderly persons with this disease, the problem is not only reduced insulin production, but also an inability to regulate glucose transport into the cells. If such individuals eat too many carbohydrates, their blood sugar rises excessively. On the other hand, if they do not eat, their blood sugar declines, resulting in cravings for chocolate and other carbohydrates. When treated with the 2-AEP complex, this phenomenon practically disappears. It is important to note that considerably increasing vitamin C intake enhances the effectiveness of the 2-AEP complex dramatically, thus allowing for even greater diabetes control.

I feel proud to have discovered a successful protection against the degenerative effects of diabetes. There are an enormous number of people in the civilized world who must seriously count on a reduced life span because of that disease. The 2-AEP complex has proven to be an outstanding medicine in the very best sense of the word. It can be taken as a preventative measure or as a treatment for an already-present illness.

There are even more benefits of the 2-AEP complex. Heart and circulatory disease can be prevented or treated with this highly useful mineral transport substance. The heart's natural pacemaker works by generating electrical impulses that ultimately produce muscular contractions of the ventricles. The contractions force blood automatically through the arteries in regular rhythmic pulses. The pacemaker system, located in the heart muscle, is not made up of nerve fibers, but rather consists of structurally and chemically modified heart muscle cells that transmit and conduct the impulses to the ventricles. A notable characteristic of the heart-rhythm cells is that they can be damaged by the impaired combustion of neutral fats, which produces an abrupt disturbance of the pacemaker system and often results in a heart attack. This damaging effect can be overcome if the necessary mineral substances for proper heart cell function are provided. These include magnesium and potassium aspartates, vitamin C, selenium, l-carnitine, and the 2-AEP complex.

Furthermore, the 2-AEP complex plays a significant role in the treatment of high blood pressure. It increases cellular membrane integrity in the cells of the heart, arteries, and blood, allowing the cells to function optimally. And by sealing the cellular membrane free-lipid pore sites (discussed on page 62), the 2-AEP complex prevents intrusion of the herpes and cytomegalo viruses into the heart and arterial cells. The latter have only recently been linked to serious heart and arterial diseases. Thus, the mineral transport substances derived from the aminoethylphosphates have extensive (in fact, overwhelming) benefits concerning our health.

From the information provided in this chapter, it is clear that the active mineral transporters are highly effective in the prevention and the treatment of many types of chronic disease. In the following chapters, I present in-depth discussions on specific diseases, beginning with what is known as the number-one killer in the United States—cardiovascular disease. With the knowledge you will gain from this information, you will further understand what you can do to enhance your quality and quantity of life.

■■■■■ CHAPTER 6 ■■■■■

*P*REVENTING AND TREATING CAR OVASCULAR EASE

Everywh   eart because its vessels run to all
his limb

from *The Beginning of the*
Secret Book of the Physician
Circa 1550 B.C.

The term *cardiovascular* refers to the heart and the blood vessels. Heart disease, stroke (cerebrovascular accident), and coronary disease are collectively referred to as *cardiovascular disease,* which affects over 65 million Americans and constitutes the leading cause of death in the United States. While many conditions are included under the label of cardiovascular disease, most of them can be traced back to arteriosclerosis and hypertension (chronic high blood pressure).

In the American population, it is estimated that cardiovascular disease is responsible for over 1 million deaths each year. Sixty million Americans suffer from hypertension.

Over 5 million have primary coronary disease and more than 2 million have had debilitating strokes. Furthermore, about 2 million Americans experience the effects of rheumatic heart disease. The statistics are frightening. Every American should learn as much as possible about cardiovascular illness—how to prevent and, if necessary, how to treat it.

ARTERIOSCLEROSIS

Arteriosclerosis, also called "hardening of the arteries," is a leading culprit of cardiovascular disease. It refers to both the loss of elasticity of the arteries—and, therefore, the decline of the arteries' ability to transport blood at a healthy blood pressure—and to the accumulation of fatty deposits in the arteries. These deposits or plaques gather along the arterial walls and narrow the vessels, also possibly resulting in increased blood pressure. In addition, the risk of clots is heightened; pieces of the deposits can break off and dangerously travel through the bloodstream, or blood corpuscles and platelets can accumulate on the plaques and block the arteries even further.

I have found that arteriosclerosis is not *primarily* caused by high fat content in the blood, as many believe. It is more often brought about by underlying inflammation processes resulting from viral infection of the blood vessel walls. Besides constricting the vessels, these inflammatory processes also interfere with *transit*—the nutrient exchange from blood to tissue.

Of course, keep in mind that diet and nutrition are at the foundation of every approach to a healthier heart. A low-fat, low-salt diet is important. Saturated fats heighten the possibility of plaque accumulations in the arteries, and excess sodium puts strain on the circulatory system. Then there are a number of additional approaches to treating and/or preventing arteriosclerosis.

Conventional Therapies for Arteriosclerosis

Conventional therapies for arteriosclerosis generally attack the problem after it has become severe. In my opinion, they do not aim at the source of the problem. However, the advanced surgical techniques of orthodox medicine have helped extend the lives of many individuals. On the other hand, conventional treatment approaches also encourage taking medications that enhance blood circulation, but these medications are often merely of brief value. Orthodox approaches are discussed below.

Surgery

To combat advanced arteriosclerosis, orthodox medicine utilizes surgery. Either blockages in vessels are by-passed with portions of healthier vessels from elsewhere in the body, or laser surgery is used to disintegrate plaques. However, there is always considerable risk with these methods (especially risks of traveling clots), and recovery time is quite long. Many people do not respond well to the aggressiveness of this approach. If surgery is necessary and ultimately successful, cardiologists feel that the benefits last approximately ten years, but every individual is different. So in cases where immediate intervention is not required, it is best to consider alternative options.

Clofibrate Compounds

Orthodox medicine also suggests the use of clofibrate compounds, which are synthetic (not natural to the body) substances. While clofibrates reduce blood-fat levels, they are essentially a cosmetic treatment. They do not improve blood vessel elasticity, which should be the essential criterion for success. Actually, the clofibrates produce a tendency towards a fatty liver and can reinforce *angina pectoris* attacks, which are attacks of chest pain due to lack of sufficient oxygen in the heart muscle. Clofibrate therapy was prohibited in Germany by the Federal Health Authority in 1976, but later it was partly readmitted.

Statins

In the late 1970s, the statins—Simavastatin; Fluvastatin; Lovastatin; and the most aggressive, Carivastatin—were introduced for the treatment of *hyperlipidemia*, which is the presence of excess fats (lipids) in the blood. Again, in this type of therapy, the main focus is on reducing blood-fat levels. The long-term effects of the statins have not been very positive. As a matter of fact, the statins are reported to create a series of severe problems in the liver and heart muscle, where they inhibit the formation of life-essential *quinones*—important coenzymes that catalyze several biological processes.

Alternative Therapies for Arteriosclerosis

There is a major contrast between the agendas of orthodox medicine and those of modern alternative medicine. Alternative approaches endeavor to correct the problem at its most basic beginnings, not merely to remove the problem once it has severely advanced.

Bromelain

Prevention of arteriosclerosis plays a significant role in increasing life expectancy. For this purpose, alternative orthomolecular therapy promotes the enzyme bromelain (natural to pineapples and other fruits and vegetables), which is absorbed into the bloodstream and can be used without limitation. This approach is as effective after eight year's use as it is on the first day. Bromelain cleans blood vessel walls and cells, and dissolves already-existing clots. So it has an excellent cleaning effect on arterial deposits. (Its actions are comparable to the long-term use of magnesium orotate, discussed in Chapter 5.) Bromelain is taken in pill form. The most effective bromelain preparations are those that include a number of additional food enzymes, among which are amylase, chymotrypsin, lipase, pancreatin, papain, protease, rutin, and trypsin. I have gained much of my information on bromelain from the work of Dr. Steven Taussig of Honolulu, Hawaii, who is responsible for a very large amount of research on this substance.

Interestingly, in performing extensive cancer therapy, I have found that bromelain unmasks the surface antigens of malignant cells, thus allowing them to be recognized by the body's lymphocytes and macrophages (important components of the natural immune defense system). And among the many cancer patients whom I have treated, there have been a number with angina pectoris. Almost from the very start of the bromelain cancer therapy, the angina pectoris largely regressed in these patients.

Chelation Therapy

In both the United States and Germany, chelation therapy with EDTA (ethylene diamine tetra-acetic acid)—a substance that removes toxic heavy metals from the body and indirectly dissolves the calcium out of deposits—is used successfully by alternative practitioners for the treatment of arteriosclerosis. Chelation agents are soluble organic compounds that can scavenge certain metallic ions into their molecular structure, allowing them to be excreted in the urine. EDTA and most other chelating agents are taken orally, but may also be injected intramuscularly (IM).

Ozone

One of the strongest treatments available for the immediate reduction of general inflammation is ozone. Ozone (O_3) is created when oxygen (O_2) is exposed to ultraviolet rays, which occurs naturally in the upper levels of the earth's atmosphere. It has powerful oxidizing properties and is a very effective antiseptic and disinfectant, thus turning harmful chemicals and elements into nontoxic substances. Among its many uses, ozone can be given intravenously to reduce circulatory problems and promote oxygen production in the body's tissues. Furthermore, it enhances the immune system to further fight disease. So this treatment, considered an alternative therapy, is recognized as a significant therapy for cardiovascular disease.

CLOTS AND RESULTING TISSUE DESTRUCTION

Thrombosis—undesirable clotting in the blood vessels—can occur due to inflammation of the veins, as well as to electrical membrane changes in red blood corpuscles and platelets. Thrombosis can also be the result of the build-up of plaques in the vessels. As deposits increase in size, it is possible that pieces will break off and dangerously travel through the bloodstream. It is also possible that corpuscles and platelets will catch on the plaques along vessel walls and accumulate, causing further obstruction in the artery. A *heart attack* occurs when the heart tissue suddenly dies because a *thrombus* (stationary clot) or an *embolism* (traveling clot that eventually lodges in a vessel that is too narrow to pass through) blocks blood flow and deprives an area of oxygen and other nutrients. A *stroke* takes place in the brain, and is also due to tissue damage/death as a result of a clot, or possibly by the breaking of a vessel.

Conventional Therapies for Clots

Orthodox medicine has several approaches to the prevention and treatment of clots. To reduce the risk of clotting, orthodox cardiology offers *anticoagulants*, such as Coumadin. These substances are preventative. They have no effect against already-existing clots, and little effect on the surface of red blood corpuscles and platelets (thrombocytes). Furthermore, anticoagulants have only a limited effect against already-existing deposits and inflammations along the vein walls, and even less effect on the arterial walls. Anticoagulants essentially thin the blood. If an individual on this type of medication is cut, profuse bleeding can occur. The use of such medications must be carefully monitored by a physician.

In special cases, orthodox medicine offers a bacterial enzyme called *streptokinase* to dissolve thrombi. However, it is very expensive and useful for only a limited period of time. Like Coumadin and other anticoagulants, it requires very close and careful laboratory control and physician monitoring.

Alternative Therapy for Clots

Alternative orthomolecular medicine uses bromelain, discussed previously regarding the treatment of arteriosclerosis, to prevent and treat clotting. Remember, the body does not build up a resistance to bromelain. This natural, harmless substance dissolves already-existing clots and cleans blood vessel walls and cells.

HEART ATTACK

Of all the forms of cardiovascular disease, heart attack is the most feared, for it is sudden and often devastating. As defined previously, a heart attack is the sudden death of heart tissue as a result of oxygen deprivation to the heart muscle. Heart attack can be caused by a number of factors, including arteriosclerosis. But recently, research has turned to common household detergents as the responsible factor in the sharp rise in the number of fatal heart attacks.

Detergents' Harmful Effects

Over the last fifty years, the number of heart attacks in the developed nations has increased over eight-fold. Kern Wildenthal, MD, a leading cardiologist at the Heart Center of the University of Texas at Dallas, has stated that the increase in fatal heart attacks may be correlated with the use of household detergents, especially those used for dishwashing in private homes. When compared with less-developed countries, developed nations use profuse amounts of chemical detergents in their homes.

Wildenthal's study, published in the German journal *Arztliche Praxis* in 1978, reports that in the eastern European countries, the frequency of fatal heart attacks did not increase until modern lifestyles, including the use of manufactured cleaning products, were adopted. It follows that the rise in frequency of fatal heart attacks occurred primarily in the cities where these manufactured detergent substances were available, rather than in the rural areas. This situation was also found to be true in Japan.

But the most convincing evidence is found in Dr. Wildenthal's report concerning some of the oil-rich Arabs in Kuwait who have built new houses equipped with the latest kitchen equipment and dishwashers. Among this small population group, the people have had a sharp increase in the level of blood triglycerides (neutral fats) and an increase in the incidence of heart attacks. The bulk of Kuwait's population still lives a very simple lifestyle in the desert and cleans their dishes with sand. The group who continues the traditional lifestyle is characterized by very low blood-fat levels and hardly any heart attacks. The difference cannot be attributed to diet, because the wealthy Kuwaitis' eating habits are nearly the same as the traditional desert peoples', as both groups follow the same religious dietary laws. Detergents are again suspected to be the key factor.

In studying this issue, I have found that during water shortages, people with dishwashers reduce their rinsing cycles and consequently display extremely high levels of neutral fats in their blood. In November 1982, German Public Television (ARD) aired a program on the damaging effects of detergents and surfactants on plants and small animals. We are no exception. It is evident that an increase in neutral fats is closely associated with high heart attack risk. Importantly, the heart muscle is not in jeopardy because diet has resulted in a great increase of neutral fats in the blood; *rather, blood fats are high because combustion of these fats in the heart has been impaired or impeded.* The heart muscle can and must obtain up to 48 percent of its energy through the combustion of fat. The process of fatty-acid combustion in the heart muscle is easily impaired by several environmental poisons, certain medications, and several immune-blocking processes. What can we do to help our bodies combust neutral fats more efficiently? The answer is found in the arginates.

The Helpful Effects of the Arginates

Based upon a survey of millions of patients, Dr. B. Lubec has reported that type II diabetes reduces life expectancy by about eight years, mostly through fatal heart attacks and cardiovascular failure. Orthodox medicine uses sulfonyl urea (glibinclamid) to control type II diabetes. My staff and I have found that this substance does not sufficiently control the disease, however, and it has potentially serious side effects. So, instead, we promote the nontoxic orthomolecular arginates. They are far more effective in the treatment of type II diabetes, and they have no side effects!

In 1973, my staff at Hannover and I received an important grant from the Volkswagen Foundation to investigate hyperlipidemia, fatty liver, and late-onset type II diabetes. Upon clinical observation, we found a dramatic rise in the number of type II diabetes cases in the developed industrial countries—from almost none in 1960, to more than thirteen times the prevalence of type I diabetes at the present time. In compatibility with Dr. Wildenthal's study on detergents, we were able to conclude that this rise is almost exclusively related to the introduction and widespread use of detergents for dishwashing.

Recently, an *electric snake molecule* has been identified.
Under the influence of insulin, this molecule regulates the
glucose transport into our cells. The electric-chain nature of
this molecule makes it extremely sensitive to even the
smallest trace of detergent. We have found that the glu-
cose-accepting site of our cells is an *arginate* with a positive
electrical charge. As Chapter 5 explains, the late Dr. Franz
Kohler and I designed arginate mineral transporters. Since
1996, these arginate mineral transporters have become our
most advanced tool in the fight against type II diabetes.
Very small daily quantities (about 2.5 grams) of magnesium and calcium arginates significantly reduce blood glucose in individuals with type II diabetes and restore the
effectiveness of insulin, thus allowing the body to maintain
blood glucose at a desired level. I consider this to be one of
my most significant clinical research discoveries. As diabetes becomes better managed, the prevalence of cardiovascular disease is ultimately indirectly reduced through
the use of these arginate therapies.

AVAILABLE AVENUES TO CARDIOVASCULAR HEALTH

In addition to the alternative treatments that I have discussed above, my colleagues and I use several safe and
effective ways to increase the health of the cardiovascular
system. They are based on substances that the body naturally possesses and to which our systems naturally
respond.

Carnitine

Around 1960, the French pharmacist Renier, a close collaborator of my colleague Dr. Henri Laborit of Paris, published a very interesting report on the effect of *l*-carnitine,
an important amino acid that occurs naturally in the liver.
Carnitine improves the combustion of fatty acids and thus

releases more energy to the heart muscles. Fifteen years later, the Italians started using carnitine to treat children whose lives were in jeopardy due to a defect in their ability to carry out essential fatty acid combustion (beta oxidation). This therapy prevented serious heart degeneration and failure.

I routinely administer carnitine, along with magnesium orotate, to my heart patients. This combination maintains the functional health of the heart and circulatory system. Carnitine transports fatty acids to the cellular mitochondria within the heart cells, enabling the heart to obtain its necessary energy. I have found that supplementing intensive carnitine therapy with vitamin B_1 greatly enhances its effect.

Today, there is an ever-increasing interest in taking carnitine as part of a dietary supplement routine. It is now also known to dramatically reduce cholesterol deposits from the vascular system, and to clean up fatty deposits in the heart.

Potassium-Magnesium Aspartate

In 1958, guided by the earlier work of Drs. Hans Selye of Montreal and S. von Nida of Munich, I succeeded in developing potassium-magnesium aspartate as an active mineral transport system that effectively restores magnesium and potassium to the cells of the heart. Concurrently in Paris, Dr. Henri Laborit developed the same active transport molecule, as discussed in Chapter 5. We were both granted patents.

In 1962, I demonstrated before the German Society of Cardiovascular Diseases that potassium-magnesium aspartate protects the heart and liver from degeneration and collapse in the absence of sufficient oxygen. It does so through the formation of energy-rich phosphates, especially adenosinetriphosphate (ATP), which provides much needed energy and oxygen to the blood. This ATP-energy becomes paramount in overcoming the risk of cardiac cellular necrosis or destruction, coronary thrombosis, arteriosclerosis, and, most importantly, cardiac arrest. Potassium-magnesium aspartate was introduced to Germany and Japan in 1964 to 1965. Since then, through studies performed in those countries, we have found that potassium-magnesium aspartate reduces the occurrence of secondary heart attacks by about 90 percent in non-diabetic patients who are correctly treated over a continuous period of time. Incidentally, the orotates produce the same results.

Today, potassium-magnesium aspartate is an essential element in my successful treatment of cardiovascular disease and particularly in the prevention of secondary heart attacks. It is marketed worldwide, prescribed mostly by doctors but also available as an over-the-counter health product. Potassium-magnesium aspartate is now one of the most widely used heart "medications" in the world. In fact, in Germany, potassium-magnesium aspartate has become the number one medication in the control of cardiac arrhythmia (irregular heart rhythm). This substance helps the natural pacemaker to maintain healthy function. It can be used as a preventative measure or a treatment approach.

Selenium

The function of the heart's pacemaker system is quite similar to the electrical distributor of an automobile engine. This rhythm system of the heart muscle does not consist of nerve fibers, but rather of structurally and chemically modified heart muscle cells that control the heart's impulse transmission and conduction. This system is very resistant to a lack of oxygen in the blood. In fact, it can continue to be active even after clinical death.

For the heart patient facing serious pacemaker problems, there is great value in the prudent use of selenium therapy, particularly when combined with glutathione (a widely occurring peptide of amino acids) or its precursor, acetyl-cysteine. This combination inactivates free radicals in the body; removes heavy metals such as lead; serves as a potent antiviral and anticancer agent; and prevents heart damage. Following a twenty-year observation study that my colleagues and I conducted at our clinic, we have concluded that selenium particularly benefits the heart's natural pacemaker system and greatly reduces heart-rhythm disturbances. The incidence of acute cardiac arrest is almost totally eliminated when selenium and glutathione are taken together. At the other end of the spectrum, a serious selenium deficiency could lead to death of a portion of the heart muscle due to insufficient blood supply.

The past few years have brought a growing recognition of the value of selenium, a trace mineral, despite the frequent warnings from orthodox practitioners that selenium is "poisonous." Of course, in extreme overdose, this mineral is toxic, as is too much champagne, sugar, and roast beef. But if taken wisely under a health professional's supervision, selenium is highly beneficial. The therapeutic question is: How much selenium, or what blood level of selenium, is safely considered sufficient? Professor G. Schrauzer of the University of Southern California at La Jolla determined the amount of selenium needed by the body as 150 to 160 micrograms per liter (mcg/l) of blood serum. Orthodox medicine claims these standards are extreme. In my opinion, Schrauzer's suggested requirement is realistic. (For information on selenium deficiency and viruses, see page 83.)

Serrapeptase

I have found serrapeptase to be an extraordinary substance for safely removing fibrous blockages from coronary arteries, particularly the carotid arteries found in the neck, which supply blood to the brain. Serrapeptase is a natural enzyme produced by *serratia bacteria* living in silkworms. Once the silkworm has completed its transformation into a butterfly, it uses this substance to "melt" a hole in its cocoon, so that it can escape. Miniscule amounts of this enzyme are unbelievably powerful and have shown a lasting effect.

The astonishing fact is that, unlike other biological enzymes, serrapeptase affects only non-living tissue, like the silk cocoon. This is the reason the butterfly is not harmed. For our health purposes, serrapeptase dissolves only dead tissue such as the old fibrous layers that clog the lining of our arteries and dangerously restrict the flow of blood and oxygen to the brain. Because of this, serrapeptase is extremely useful in keeping arterial deposits from building up again after angioplasty (a balloon technique used to clear an artery of blockage) or coronary bypass surgery has been performed.

Very often, surgeons are reluctant or unable to open partially closed carotid arteries using laser surgery. They fear that resulting debris could be pushed into the smaller connecting arteries and result in a stroke and possibly death. In cases of severe arterial narrowing, I have used serrapeptase with excellent, even life-saving results. Only three tablets a day over a minimum period of twelve to eighteen months are adequate to produce results. Many of my patients have shown significantly improved blood flow through their previously constricted arteries, as confirmed by ultrasound examination. Unfortunately, orthodox cardiologists do not employ this important method in their practices.

The Takeda Company in Japan is the major commercial manufacturer of the serratia bacterial cultures and the largest producer of this miracle enzyme. Although it is also excellent for the treatment of swellings, it is not as effective as bromelain in the treatment of phlebitis (vein inflammation) and newly formed clots.

Calcium, Magnesium, Potassium 2-Aminoethylphosphate (2-AEP Complex; Colamine Phosphate Complex)

Calcium, magnesium, potassium 2-aminoethylphosphate, also referred to as the 2-AEP complex and the colamine phosphate complex, is an essential substance required to maintain the structural integrity of all cellular membranes. It is particularly important to the membranes of our blood and heart-muscle cells. As explained in Chapter 5 (pages 65 to 67), the 2-AEP complex seals the free-lipid pore sites in cellular membranes, preventing penetration by toxins, bacteria, and viruses that may produce serious cardiovascular disease.

VIRUSES AND CARDIOVASCULAR DISEASE

Only recently have viruses and superviruses been implicated in cardiovascular and other major chronic diseases. Significant evidence has been presented by Robert A. Sinnott, PhD, confirming the long-suspected role of herpes viruses in the most deadly and debilitating diseases of our time, including heart disease, cancer, multiple sclerosis, lupus, and Alzheimer's disease. Dr. Sinnott's findings have been published in the February 1998 edition of *Health Sciences Institute Members Alert*.

Dr. Orville Levander, with the United States Department of Agriculture (USDA), and Dr. Melinda Beck at the University of North Carolina have clearly shown that deficiencies in selenium and vitamin E can cause permanent genetic changes in the coxsackie virus, which annually affects over 20 million American children. This virus causes colds, sore throats, and diarrhea. In a selenium-deficient state, the coxsackie virus may be transformed from a benign virus into a far more virulent form that can attack the heart of infected individuals and even cause death. Incidentally, it has also been discovered that selenium deficiencies are common among AIDS (acquired immune deficiency syndrome) patients, and that supplementing selenium in patients with HIV (human immunodeficiency virus) infections increases natural immunity and delays the onset of AIDS.

The cytomegalo virus (CMV), a member of the herpes family of viruses, also has been strongly linked to heart and coronary disease. In 1997, Dr. Samuel Epstein of New York discovered that the cytomegalo virus in heart patients was responsible for blocking the action of a vital growth-limiting protein identified as p-53. The function of the p-53 protein is to prevent excessive post-surgical tissue growth within arteries following angioplasty and at coronary bypass surgical sites. When the cytomegalo virus blocks the p-53 protein action, the tissues at the surgical site or within the lining of the arteries continue their growth and, over an eight- to ten-year period, seriously restrict the normal blood flow through these arteries.

The link between viruses and chronic disease is not limited to cardiovascular illness. For some time now, I have contended that there can be no malignancy—no cancer—in the absence of the herpes I and II, varicella (chickenpox), cytomegalo, or Epstein-Barr viruses. All of these are classified as part of the herpes simplex virus family. The origin of many other chronic diseases, such as Lou Gehrig's disease (amyotrophic lateral sclerosis), multiple sclerosis, neurodermatitis, psoriasis, pulmonary fibrosis, Bell's palsy, colitis, chronic rheumatism, and many more, can also be traced directly to these viruses. It has become evident that Dr. Israel Davidson, one of the greatest American researchers, and the outstanding French researcher Dr. Oberling were correct in their assertion that *there are no chronic diseases other than those induced by herpes viruses or their sub-component infections, and their period of latency can extend for twenty years or more.* To confirm the role of viruses in chronic disease, I have shown that inactivating the herpogenic virus factor within the infected cell's mito-chondrial membrane leads to regression of disease. Our understanding of chronic disease mechanisms must be deeply reconsidered in light of these new findings.

THE FINNISH STUDY OF ORTHODOX CARDIOLOGY

A dramatic shock occurred in the world of orthodox cardi-ology when a paper from Finland, written by Strandberg and his coauthors, was published in the *Journal of the American Medical Association (JAMA)* in 1991. The article on this Helsinki research discusses a long-term study of more than 1,200 patients exhibiting "high heart attack risks," such as hypertension, high levels of blood lipids (fats), anginal pain, diabetes, and earlier cardiac tissue failure. More than half of these patients received a full complement of conventional cardiac treatment, including: diuretics; anti-lipid medications like clofibrate and Lovastatin; nitrates; antihypertensive drugs; and calcium antagonists such as Nifidipin. To provide a control group, about 45 per-cent of the participants did not receive any therapy at all.

After seven years, the group who had been convention-ally treated performed slightly better with respect to sur-vival rate and the reduction of recurrent heart attacks than the untreated control group. However, the study was con-tinued for another ten years. The result was shocking: When compared with the survival rate of the untreated group, twice as many individuals in the therapeutic group died in this time period.

Since 1991, documentation has been sent to all doctors informing them of the "collapse" of conventional ap-proaches to cardiac therapy. I find the Finnish report to be of great interest for the following reason: The biological organ-ism profits from orthodox toximolecular drugs for only a limited period. Over time, the organism becomes increas-ingly resistant to substances that are alien to its natural biochemical and biophysical system. The conclusions that must be drawn from this may indeed apply to all avenues of the orthodox medical treatment of chronic disease. They explain why orthodox toximolecular treatments do not result in a real increase in life expectancy, very much in contrast to the results obtained from alternative orthomolecular medicine and natural biological therapies.

As this chapter indicates, it is important that we take preventative measures to combat cardiovascular disease. And if disease is already present, it is important to consider *all* of the treatment options, even those that aren't promoted by the conventional healthcare industry. Moreover, be suspect of orthodox therapies that make big promises but, in the long run, yield small results. Orthomolecular approaches to chronic disease are now surfacing as the more promising, more beneficial avenues of treatment. Further support for the orthomolecular approaches regarding chronic disease can be found in alternative cancer treatments, as the next chapter will discuss.

CHAPTER 7

$\mathcal{D}$ETECTING AND TREATING CANCER

Much of what is done in the treatment of cancer . . . is directed at the existence of already established cancer cells, but not at the mechanisms by which cells become neoplastic.

from *The Lives of a Cell*
—Dr. Lewis Thomas (b. 1913)

With the same spirit of hope and drive as it puts forth to find treatments for cardiovascular disease, today's medical research community is urgently searching to find effective cures for cancer. Cancer has afflicted man since he first walked on earth. Indeed, Cro-Magnon man is thought to have died from cancer.

We know that cancer is not a disease that can be considered "under control," for its incidence continues to rise. It appears that some naturally occurring phenomenon determines whether a patient will develop a malignancy or not, and little progress has been made toward revealing the causative processes of cancer and providing effective protection. Current orthodox cancer therapies—surgery, chemotherapy, and radiation—most often fail to save the patient. But alternative, orthomolecular treatment approaches are changing that dismal outlook.

DEFINING CANCER AND ITS CAUSES

Cancer is best described as the uncontrolled growth of abnormal cells. It can occur in any tissue or organ of the body. As the number of cancerous cells increases, a malignant mass called a *tumor* forms. The tumor often infests surrounding tissue. It is likely that one or more cancer cells will break away from the parent tumor and invade tissues or organs in other areas of the body, thus spreading the cancer. These secondary cancers are called *metastases*, or *metastatic growths*. Unchecked cancerous growths (both primary and secondary) interfere with the body's ability to function, resulting in extreme illness and, frequently, death.

There are well over 100 different types of cancer. Each may be pathologically classified into one of five major groups: *carcinoma*, a cancerous growth of the mucous membrane or epithelial tissues; *sarcoma*, a malignant solid tumor of the muscle, bone, or connective tissue; *leukemia*, an uncontrolled proliferation of the leukocytes (a type of white blood cell); *lymphoma*, a malignant tumor of the lymphatic tissue or lymph nodes; and *myeloma*, a malignancy of plasma cells stemming from the bone marrow.

Our bodies constantly combat abnormal cells. A healthy immune system can kill off a cancerous cell before multiplication and a resulting growth occur. However, our immune systems cannot catch and disable *every* abnormality within the body. And then there are several key factors that influence immunity and our bodies' general protective functions.

Diet

Twenty-four hours a day, a person is under the influence of what he or she eats. Diet is a major factor in the development of cancer. I must stress that diet is fundamental to the prevention, treatment, and control of cancer. Any physician stating otherwise should be disqualified as a suitable health counselor.

High-fat, low-fiber diets increase the risk of colon cancer and are clearly implicated in prostate and breast cancer, as well as in heart disease. Meat, sausage, dairy, and cheese products should be strenuously avoided, since they increase the production of immune-blocking mucous. Shellfish should also be avoided because its high concentration of nucleic acids can be cancer-activating. Also, heavy alcohol consumption has been closely associated with mouth and throat cancer.

The immune system cannot be sustained by a diet of devitalized foods. I strongly advise a diet based on millet and enzyme-rich foods, which are quite helpful in slowing down the progress of cancer. Unprocessed living plants— fresh fruits and vegetables—contain all of the essential nutrients necessary for good health. Processing or cooking them destroys many of their essential elements. Raw or lightly cooked vegetables provide the natural enzymes, vitamins, and many of the minerals fundamental to a healthy immune system.

It has been shown that foods rich in vitamin A guard against chemical carcinogenesis—that is, the initial development of cancer due to toxic chemicals. Vitamin C promotes healing and the building of strong collagen—the "glue" that binds us together. Natural riboflavin and nicotinamide increase cellular oxidation. Riboflavin, also known as vitamin B_2, is found in B complex supplements and a number of foods, some of which are cheese, egg yolks, fish, meat, legumes, spinach, whole grains, and yogurt. Nicotinamide, or vitamin B_3, is also found in numerous food sources, including brewer's yeast, liver, eggs, fish, milk, broccoli, potatoes, tomatoes, and whole wheat products, among many others. Supplementing an energy-rich, balanced diet with beta-carotene, calcium, selenium, magnesium, molybdenum, potassium, zinc, and vitamins C, D_2, and E is essential in promoting the strong immune system so critical in the battle against cancer.

Environment

Environmental factors have a very strong influence on the body's tendency to develop cancer. Some environmental agents linked to the development of cancer include polluted water; chemical, biological, and nuclear waste; pesticides; airborne pollutants; asbestos; and radiation. Specifically, exposure to excessive electromagnetic radiation from electrical transformer banks, high-tension transmission lines, and the earth's geopathic zones has been linked to leukemia and brain tumors. (The geopathic zones are areas in which changes in the earth's magnetic field produce abnormally high concentrations of magnetic flux or energy. This change in magnetism affects our bodies at the cellular level.)

Cigarette smoke is a significant environmental carcinogen. Smokers have a high incidence of lung cancer, and even second-hand smoke is known to be associated with lung cancer. Also, detergents and other solvents and aromatics (halogenated hydrocarbons) contribute to the development of cancer. Industrial pollution and auto/bus exhaust are thought to be major contributors to serious chronic diseases, including cancer. The incidence of lung cancer is much greater in major metropolitan areas than in farming areas.

However, the incidence of skin cancer is much greater in rural areas and in beach areas, where people are more exposed to damaging ultraviolet (UV) energy from the sun. Also, certain geographic areas, such as Australia, are experiencing dramatic increases in skin cancer and melanoma possibly due to holes in the protective ozone layer. These holes allow greater amounts of ultraviolet radiation to penetrate to the earth's surface. But in addition, the high incidence of skin cancer in Australia is due to the fact that fair-skinned people only recently immigrated to that part of the world. The generations born of these blood lines are not genetically prepared for the intense radiation from the sun.

Heredity

There appear to be genetic predispositions to cancer that run through family lines. Breast cancer is an example of a type of cancer that seems to have a strong hereditary link. In cases of hereditary cancer, there may be actual transmission of genetically altered cells (the sperm or the ova is altered), or there may be transmission of latent viral DNA passed on from generation to generation. Also, there could be defects in hereditary immune genes.

Stress

It is not uncommon that after an individual experiences great physiological and/or emotional stress, his or her immune system is suppressed. As a result, some cells may begin to grow at an unchecked rate. This uncontrollable cell growth produces cancer. Therefore, it is important to learn stress-management techniques for the inevitable pressures that you face, and to avoid stressful environments whenever possible.

Considering the fast pace of today's world, it would do all of us well to concentrate on providing ourselves with frequent mental and physical relaxation. Furthermore, if you have suffered tremendous loss and grief, it is important to manage these psychological stresses through good counseling. Emotional depression leads to physical depression, primarily the depression of the immune system.

ORTHODOX CANCER THERAPY

In order to better control cancer, it is necessary to become more acquainted with how the healthy body daily prohibits cancer from developing, and then to imitate that mechanism. Unfortunately, orthodox medicine has not taken this approach. Instead, it aims only to remove evident cancer and to kill affected and/or possibly affected tissue, in the hopes that all traces of the disease will be eliminated. Orthodox approaches—surgery, chemotherapy, and radiation therapy—address the symptoms, not the underlying biological, genetic, and/or viral causes. They don't teach the body, itself, to fight cancer. These treatments are, at best, short-term methods, albeit sometimes successful.

Surgery

Quite obviously and simply, surgery aims to cut out the area of cancerous growth. Many cancer patients have operations in which cancerous tumors are completely removed. Then, knowing that their bodies have been victim to cancer cells, these patients must monitor themselves carefully for any recurrence. For example, a woman with advanced cancer in her breast can have the breast completely removed through an operation called a *mastectomy*. Physicians will also look at surrounding lymph nodes, hopefully identifying any metastases, and will often remove any nodes that are potentially cancerous. Once the surgery is performed, this woman's treatment is not over. She will most likely endure follow-up radiation or chemotherapy sessions and will be closely and regularly watched for any evidence of recurrence, as she is considered to be at increased risk.

At least surgical intervention does not damage the patient's immune defense mechanisms. However, the patient is not "cured" by the radical nature of the surgery. A cure happens only when the internal defense mechanism gains and maintains the upper hand over the multiplication of cancerous cells.

Chemotherapy

Chemotherapy involves the use of a specific chemical agent or agents to arrest the progress of cancer or to destroy a cancerous growth, hopefully without causing irreversible damage to the majority of healthy cells. Most chemotherapeutic agents are simply normal cellular "nutrients" (metabolites) that have been chemically altered by adding a poisonous atom or atoms to the nutrient's molecular structure. Such an alteration renders the substance a highly toxic, potent anticancer agent. One example is uracil plus a fluorine atom, yielding 5-Fluorouracil (5-FU), a widespread agent for the orthodox treatment of cancer that was discovered during testing under an American Cancer Society (ACS) grant at Sloan-Kettering Institute. The ACS continues to receive 50 percent of this drug's revenue.

Because most cancer cells grow and multiply at many times the rate of normal noncancerous cells, it is expected by design that these cancer cells will compete unfairly for and will consume more of these chemotherapeutic nutrients. Hence, they will be killed at a greater differential rate than will normal cells. Unfortunately however, significant numbers of normal cells *are* destroyed by these highly toxic agents. Furthermore, toxic chemotherapy weakens and destroys the body's natural immune system and renders it incapable of effectively fighting against cancer recurrence.

Through testing on animals, the medical community established that chemotherapy is reasonably effective in controlling cancer only if the animal's defenses are not too severely damaged. Thus, the "tail wind" effect provided by the body's defenses is essential to the success of chemotherapy. In children up to about fourteen years of age, chemotherapy may be quite useful in the control of malignancies, since a young body's defense system more easily assists the chemotherapeutic effects, while disposing of the toxic aftermath.

If an individual is free from cancer for five years after chemotherapy, the ACS proclaims him or her "cured." The use of that word is rather ambiguous; it gives the patient the impression that the treatment has permanently worked, when, in reality, the cancer often returns at a later date. Chemotherapy is often defended by orthodox medicine with heated aggression. Yet this highly toxic treatment is, in fact, no better suited to cancer therapy than a zeppelin balloon would be to a massive trans-Atlantic airlift. Only a few may reach the other shore and at an enormous cost, both financially and in terms of the quality of life. I am not suggesting that chemotherapy should never be used, but it should be managed with precise balancing.

Radiation

Radiation therapy uses electromagnetic waves from naturally radioactive sources (for example, cobalt) to target and destroy a tumor by literally burning it away. Again, the principal problem is that healthy cells are also destroyed. As a result, just as in the case of chemotherapy, radiation treatment adversely affects the immune system, possibly to the point where the body cannot fight recurrence.

Patient prognosis after radiation therapy is very similar to prognosis after chemotherapy. Those who benefit most are those who come to radiation therapy with a reasonably well-functioning immune system. People who are very weak end up being further weakened by the aggressive nature of this therapy.

A Long-Term View

Orthodox medicine does not offer either preventive or adequate long-term protective therapy. Unfortunately, in most cases of radiation and sometimes chemotherapy, the disease outlasts the treatment's period of effectiveness. Ultimately, conventional medicine remains caught up in pursuing those treatments that fail to save the patient from death.

In the 1970s, deaths due to cancer numbered 350,000 annually. Today, in the United States, there is one cancer death per minute, and thus more than 500,000 deaths due to cancer per year. It is evident that in spite of advances in diagnostic techniques—the development of mammograms, MRIs, PET and CAT scans, all of which help in the earlier detection of cancer—the conventional ways of treating cancer are not making things better. Furthermore, 1 million new cancer patients were diagnosed in 1997. It is obvious that the medical community needs to add new therapies to its list of approaches.

Unfortunately, many physicians are not open to other ways of preventing and treating cancer. When a patient asks what diet should be followed, some orthodox doctors typically reply, "Eat what you want, there's no cancer diet." Or if an individual asks, "What else can I do?", the answer is often, "We've done everything possible, so you don't need to worry any further." The final advice is, "Come back in three to six months for a check-up." If patients ask about alternative medicine options, they are frequently ridiculed or told that unconventional methods are unproven remedies. I do not mean to imply that most doctors in the United States are malicious, but simply that many know so little about alternative therapies that they cannot give a truly educated opinion on them.

In truth, many alternative cancer medicines have been clinically proven and effectively used for years throughout the rest of the world. When American patients do go to other countries for alternative cancer treatment, they frequently avoid telling their oncologists. Subsequent improvement is often credited to their previous orthodox therapy, or to the miracle of "spontaneous remission."

THE IMMUNE SYSTEM AND CANCER

When the risk of cancer continues to exist, especially after a cancer operation, there are protective measures taken by the body. It is these measures that alternative medicine aims to uncover and imitate, for they work far more effectively against cancer than previously assumed. There are several important elements that make up the basic human immuno-defense system: antibodies; granulocytes and macrophages; complements; and the lymphocytes.

The *antibody system* is comprised of protein substances in the blood that are created by the body to attack and destroy foreign invaders called *antigens*. This antibody-antigen reaction is generally very specific to a certain disease. An antibody will attack only the antigen that instigated the antibody's formation.

The second line of immuno-defense in the body is the *granulocytes,* or granulated white blood cells. These cells are constantly on patrol, tirelessly searching the body for poisonous material. When granulocytes identify an invader, they mobilize millions of cells and attack relentlessly until the invader is destroyed. If the granulocytes are incapable of overcoming these invaders on their own, they call in powerful reinforcements called *macrophages,* that are larger, stronger white blood cells.

The third component of the body's immuno-defense system is the *complements*, which are groups of nine highly-specialized proteins in our blood serum that are manufactured by the liver and called into action by the antibodies. Complements are extremely aggressive and cannot always differentiate between friend and foe. They will attack normal healthy cells as quickly as they will attack poisonous invaders. Complements, therefore, require a special guidance system, which is provided by the antibodies. The antibodies attach a marker to each disease or foreign antigen, then activate the nearest passing unit of complement. The first of the complement's nine proteins attaches immediately to the antigen and signals the next protein. Each protein unit of the complement attaches itself to the antigen and, in turn, signals the next. By the time the ninth protein strikes, the invader is destroyed.

The *lymphocytes,* produced by the lymph nodes throughout the body, are a type of white blood cell that provide overall control over the entire immuno-defense system. These lymphocytes continuously cycle throughout the body, looking for invaders. When an invader is detected, the lymphocyte makes a "print" or copy of the antigen's marker and immediately carries the information to the nearest lymph node. The lymph node then alerts the entire immuno-defense system, mobilizing specific back-up systems such as the granulocytes and complements.

Our natural immune system's white blood cells, especially the lymphocytes, monocytes (the largest cells in normal blood, each having a round, oval, or indented single nucleus), and macrophages, are essential tools in the defense against cancer. But even when an immune system functions well, cancer can develop. For example, cancer cells frequently display a membrane-antigen configuration that is very similar to that of blood-type A, and therefore is not readily recognized by the immune system of the blood-type A individual. This is significant; in Germany, blood-type A patients represent 77 percent of the stomach cancer population. Something has to be done to provide addition-al protection to these patients. In this specific case, a con-tinuous intake of bromelain can be helpful. Bromelain is discussed in more detail on page 72.

Immune system lymphocytes are effective against can-cer cells only when they are present in sufficient numbers and possess an internal structure that is specifically acti-vated by the cancer cell steroids, by tumosteron, or by thy-mosterine. The latter two are initially triggered by a sub-stance called ergocalciferol, which is produced by the thy-mus gland. The lymph cell defenses require the use of additional *complements*, the chief proteins of blood plasma (previously discussed). Unfortunately, the complements are often not available in sufficient quantities, or are used up in the immune system battle against cancer cells. This is especially true when certain virus components of the her-pes group are responsible for initiating the cancerous growth.

The herpes groups of viruses have been identified as a primary underlying cause of many, if not all, human can-cers. (See pages 83 to 85 for information on viruses and chronic disease.) Most prominently, they are known to cause cervical and uterine cancers, ovarian cancers, certain lung cancers, tumors of the nose and throat, lymphomas, and clear-cell melanomas, just to name a few. Increasing the production of complements to fight these viruses is extremely important, but difficult. A general immune-enhancing substance called *gamma globulin* may be injected to reinforce the production of cancer-fighting complements. Thymus supplements are also helpful in stimulating the thymus gland's production of ergocalciferol. Alternative medicine can also provide much help. Through my clinical use of anticancer agents, I have found that zinc aspartate and magnesium aspartate promote complement production.

In fact, in the case of Hodgkin's disease, which causes progressive enlargement of the lymph nodes, zinc aspartate and magnesium aspartate are of decisive importance.

This brings us to a discussion on the newest alternative approaches to cancer, which seek to enhance the body's natural process of suppressing cancer by attacking it at the cellular and genetic levels.

GENETICS AND ALTERNATIVE CANCER TREATMENTS

For many years, I have focused on developing cancer treatments that utilize natural substances and the body's natural abilities to suppress cancer. In order to do this, I have investigated cancer down to its very beginnings, on the level of genetics. The substances that my colleagues and I have found effective actually repair or exterminate problematic genes that ultimately send harmful messages to their cells. If we can manipulate gene messages so that we can stop the uncontrolled reproduction of cancer cells, we can stop cancer right where it begins.

Spontaneous Remission

From my clinical experience, I have learned that most patients have cancer in their systems long before they exhibit any symptoms—in other words, long before the cancer is detected. I have also observed that, as mentioned previously, physical and/or emotional stress suppresses the immune system, thus making an individual more likely to develop cancer. Yet, there are instances in which a patient seems to be able to dramatically throw off an advanced, seemingly uncontrollable cancer spontaneously. After many years of study, I conclude that the normal immune response—that complex mechanism of defense that is normally activated by the onset of disease—does not play the major role in the phenomenon of spontaneous remission. Furthermore, I conclude that our immune defense may not be the main mechanism by which malignancies are continually suppressed in healthy individuals.

In cases of spontaneous remission, there are substances that inactivate, seal, or otherwise control the cancer cells' *genetic* information. These substances reverse the cancer process by removing the key from the genetic coding that is resulting in malignancy. Thus, cells are restored to normalcy. After more than four decades in the cancer field, these observations have led me to the realization that I must employ a multi-disciplinary approach of immune enhancement *and* genetic repair if I am to be successful in the prevention and treatment of cancer.

The Genetic System

The genetic system of each human cell contains approximately 2 billion base pairs of chromosomes. We are dealing with a "computer" that has an extremely high capacity of 2 billion bytes. Most of the genetic information remains secured through a sort of sealing and locking mechanism. Only a small amount of the stored information of genetic possibilities is permitted to be released. This maintains a rather uniform and healthy production of cells. In fact, it appears that the genetic system has its own special watchdog genes responsible for maintaining the proper order. Formation of the type and function of genes is pre-programmed and quite secure.

Normally, 99 percent of all carried genes is locked within the cells like data in a computer. The genes are not permitted to give any signal. However, occasionally genes may open and release a signal leading to disorder, and possibly resulting in cancer, diabetes, or other diseases. So it is of critical importance that humans and all other living organisms possess and maintain substances that constantly ensure that the genetic systems remain in stable control.

Not all cells that carry active *oncogenes*—the genetic structures that cause malignant disorders—develop into malignancies. However, in all cases of malignancy, the membranes of the mitochondria within the cellular plasma show severe deviations from normal cell structure. These deviations are called *malignolipin*. The membranes of such mitochondria also contain DNA that undergoes damage or mutation about twenty-five times more frequently than the DNA in the cell's nucleus. This strongly suggests that the mitochondria are the principal targets and/or areas of origination of malignancy.

Natural Immunity and Gene-Repair

As I look broadly at nature, I find that trees are resistant to mushrooms and other fungi, for otherwise they would not survive. Yet trees have no immune systems. How do they defend themselves? They develop protective micro-enzymes—endopeptidases and endonucleases—which work against these fungi and other aggressors. Similarly, numerous insects, like ants, are much older than humans and lack immune systems, yet are able to defend themselves from diseases. Many genetically ancient biological structures did not start with immunity in their genetic makeup. In 1957, I discovered and published that certain structures within the mitochondria of humans are very similar to the primitive fungal structures that far predate humanity. I also observed sub-cellular elements (elements that apparently pre-date modern cell substances) which come out of cells when they become cancerous. From this, I have concluded that cancer may be much older than our immune systems.

So I began to develop specific intracellular cancer therapies based upon the use of certain substances that work against fungal infections, such as thiurams and quinones. This work, in turn, led me to investigate Laetrile (the l-glucose mandelonitrile), the mandelonitriles, and the aldehydes, which also work very effectively against these subcellular, fungus-like components of the malignant cell's genetic system.

LAETRILE

Laetrile (Laevomandelonitrile), extracted from apricot pits, is one of the most powerful anticancer substances found. As discussed in Chapter 5, Laetrile is a nontoxic compound comprised of glucose, cyanic acid, and benzaldehyde. Cancer cells produce rhodanase, an enzyme, at their membrane surface. The Laetrile molecule is split by rhodanase at the cancer site and releases the cyanic acid (HCN), which is highly toxic to cancer cells. This is the mechanism by which Laetrile is an effective anticancer agent.

The Cassettis of Florence, Italy, demonstrated that Laetrile is metabolized only by tumor cells, not by normal cells. But the national authorities in the United States elected to prosecute Laetrile supporters rather than to concentrate their efforts on producing Laetrile through genetic engineering. Unfortunately, Laetrile has not been available since the mid-1970s. In Germany, I was able to use the closely related mandelonitriles synthesized for me by the late Dr. Franz Kohler to treat my cancer patients.

I have found the mandelonitriles to be among the most effective nontoxic substances for cancer treatment. Typically, they reduce already-existing tumors. This therapy, administered orally in drops, is considered to repair health at the genetic level, as well as attack and terminate already-existing cancer cells. So it can be used in prevention and treatment.

GENE-REPAIRING AND GENE-EXTINGUISHING SUBSTANCES

Since the mid-nineteenth century, much has been learned about the genesis—the beginning, the origin—of cancer. As mentioned earlier, it is now certain that during the course of cancer genesis, the membrane systems of structures inside the cells, especially those of the mitochondria, become defective. This indirectly leads to damage of the chromosomes in the cell nucleus, and the damage leads to "gene instabilities." It is possible to alter the cancer-causative genetic structure from the nuclei of cancer cells, causing them to revert to being completely normal cells.

During the process of cancer genesis, the cell loses the calcium lining of its inner membranes, as well as magnesium and potassium. As a result, the cancer cell takes in sodium, rarely found in the normal cell body; normally, potassium is found within the cell, and sodium without. When cells replace potassium with sodium, they lose their ability to function and are unable to activate immune responses to diseases, toxins, and bacteria. Ultimately, in losing its calcium supply, the cancer cell membrane also loses its characteristic electrical condenser function. In turn, the entire immuno-defense mechanism is weakened. By absorbing more sodium, the cancer cell develops an electrical behavior that places it outside of the body's defense capability.

There are over 150 chemical and biological structures presently known that possess gene-repairing, gene-extinguishing, or resistance-stimulating properties against cancer cells, degenerating cells, and certain large viruses, especially of the herpes strain. I am currently using a number of the new gene-reparative substances in the treatment of cancer, together with proven nontoxic therapies, antioxidant vitamins, minerals, and sound dietary planning, to enhance and restore my patients' disease-weakened immune systems. The most clinically effective of these gene-repair substances are: acetaldehyde; benzaldehyde; carnivorous plant extracts; DHEA; didrovaltrate (an herbal extract from the Himalayan valerian plant); the iridodials; the oncostatins; squalene (shark liver oil); and tumosterons.

Acetaldehyde

In 1974, acetaldehyde, a common chemical substance that is closely related to benzaldehyde, was identified as an anticancer substance by Dr. Ugo Ehrenfeld at the Max Planck Institute. Acetaldehyde is a common synthetic chemical substance. The Ehrenfeld program has been successfully used in the treatment and arrest of both melanomas and brain tumors, with a positive response of almost 80 percent. In my clinic, I routinely employ acetaldehyde in the treatment of melanotic melanoma (cancer in the melanin of the skin). For this specific cancer, acetaldehyde has proven to be clearly superior to benzaldehyde, discussed below.

Benzaldehyde

During the 1970s, the late Dr. Dean Burk of the National Cancer Institute in the United States expressed the opinion that benzaldehyde, a biochemical component of Laetrile (amygdalin) and the mandelonitriles, possesses active anticancer properties. I neglected the specific study of benzaldehyde, turning my attention to the mandelonitriles that Dr. Kohler had synthesized for me. But Japanese researchers worked steadily with benzaldehyde.

In 1980, the National Cancer Institute reported the excellent results obtained in Japan with benzaldehyde. Subsequently, two Japanese researchers, Drs. Matsuyuki Kochi and Setsuo Takeuchi, found that the active anticancer component in figs was benzaldehyde. These Japanese investigators presented extensive pharmacological and clinical evidence of the effectiveness of benzaldehyde in treating a broad spectrum of cancers.

Benzaldehyde exerts a gene-extinguishing effect on the ability of cancer cells to reproduce. The good news is that normal cells are totally unaffected by benzaldehyde, there is a notable reduction in the patient's pain, and there are no toxic side effects from benzaldehyde's use as an anticancer agent. From my clinical observations, I have concluded that the least we can expect from the use of benzaldehyde as an anticancer agent is that it will arrest tumor growth for an indefinite period, allowing a complementary immune-enhancing therapy to firmly arrest the cancer.

Carnivorous Plant Extracts

Carnivorous plant extracts—for example, those derived from the carnivorous Venus fly trap plant—contain the active enzymes *endopeptidase* and *endonuclease*. These are special gene-eliminating substances. Carnivorous plant extracts eliminate malignant cells by extinguishing their genetic replication. They are also useful in eliminating tissue damaged by radiation therapy; while having no effect on normal cells. In addition, almost a dozen gene-defect-extinguishing substances in these plants, such as *plumbagin*, *droseron*, and *hydroxydroseron*, have now been identified. These substances contain special enzymes that are highly active against tumor cells and cells damaged by radiation.

Carnivorous plant extracts have been found to be very effective in the treatment of Hodgkin's disease, specific melanomas, lymphatic leukemias, and metastasizing colon carcinomas. Moreover, the administration of a carnivorous extract by intramuscular injection is extremely helpful in the treatment of herpes and similar viruses. Through inhalation therapy, carnivora extracts may be introduced into the air cells of the lungs and subsequently absorbed into the bloodstream, where they become effective anticancer agents.

Dehydroepiandrosterone (DHEA)

Dehydroepiandrosterone, commonly known as DHEA, is a steroid that was identified in Germany in 1930. It was found that *carbon disulfide*, a chemical in the atmosphere, reduces the frequency of cancer and causes the increased

activation of certain steroids, including DHEA, to be produced by the body's suprarenal gland. DHEA is present in
the blood in fairly high concentrations; it is freely floating
in the blood, not enclosed within the blood cells. DHEA is
an ever-present and very effective monitor for cancer. This
steroid increases the level of the enzyme *cholinesterase*. The
higher the level of cholinesterase, the greater the degree of
cancer regression.

During the 1970s, Dr. Arthur Schwartz, at Temple
University in Philadelphia, Pennsylvania, found that
DHEA inhibits the action of a cancer-promoting enzyme
(G6PDH). This dangerous enzyme actually converts dormant carcinogens (cancer-producing substances) into extremely active ones. DHEA is the ultimate antioxidant, preventing the formation of disease and cancer-causing free
radicals. Dr. Schwartz concluded that DHEA apparently
inhibits the cancer process by blocking the genetic action of
a variety of tumor-promoting initiators, such as ultraviolet
light from the sun, tobacco, heavy metals, fats, alcohol, and
radiation. Furthermore, in 1983, Schwartz demonstrated
that DHEA alone can stop the formation of breast cancer in
a strain of cancer-prone mice.

As people pass middle age, the amount of DHEA steadily decreases and should be supplemented. This also occurs
as cancer progresses, providing an early diagnostic marker
for the onset of the disease. As cancer advances, the DHEA
becomes used up and is not replaced. Fortunately, a combination of squalene (discussed later) and vitamin C ascorbates enhances the formation of the body's own DHEA
quite markedly. DHEA is also available as a supplement,
obtained from plant hormones.

Didrovaltrate

The valerian plant (not a carnivorous plant), which grows
high in the Himalayan mountains where it is exposed to

ultraviolet light, produces a gene-repair substance called didrovaltrate. The gene-repairing effect of this substance was first discovered by a French pharmacologist, Dr. Anton, from Strassburg. Purely by chance, a research group at the University of Strassburg, France, found that didrovaltrate was highly active against experimental Krebbs ascites breast cancer in the mouse. It is amazing to see how effective this substance is in destroying these ascites cancer cells in the mouse, specifically without harming normal cells. Didrovaltrate's molecular structure is larger but very similar to that of the iridodials (discussed later).

Based on these findings, I treated several of my cancer patients in Germany with didrovaltrate. At first, I was skeptical because the effects were not terribly dramatic. However, after one to two years, I revised my opinion and used didrovaltrate quite successfully throughout the 1980s. I found that it is particularly useful against kidney tumors and tumors of the oral cavity.

I have learned that didrovaltrate must first be changed metabolically in the patient's digestive system into an effective chemical *dialdehyde*, which, as a lipid-soluble agent, can penetrate the lipid membranes of the outer cells of large tumors. During therapy, it is necessary to administer twelve to twenty tablets (600 to 1,000 milligrams) per day, which becomes difficult for the patient to tolerate over a long period of time. Unfortunately, because no other route of administration has been found, I now employ didrovaltrate only sparingly.

The Iridodials

The iridodials are a primary source of dialdehydes, which are extremely powerful genetic-repair factors. Their anti-malignant, genetic-repair properties were first described by Dr. Peter Thies of Hannover, Germany, in 1985, and the first pulmonary tumor regression from iridodial use was observed by Dr. Didier of Gifhorn, Germany.

The iridodials are extracts obtained in extremely small yields from *iridomyrmex ants*. Insects, and particularly ants, have the capacity to produce large amounts of gene-repair substances efficiently. The result is that such insects rarely develop tumors and are able to host unbelievable amounts of viruses without showing any ill effects. Yet they have no immune systems! Since iridomyrmex ants are almost always found in geopathic zones (areas of intensely strong geomagnetic radiation), they apparently require especially strong genetic-repair systems. The iridodials are activated by the amount of geomagnetic and vacuum field energy stimulation that the ants receive.

In my clinical experience, I have observed that the iridodials outdistance most other therapeutic substances known in the treatment of cancer. They are extremely effective, even in terminal breast cancer cases, as long as the tumor has not grown beyond a certain size. These substances can be administered orally, intravenously, or intramuscularly. Not only are the iridodials more effective and much less expensive than other anticancer agents, but they are non-toxic and can be used without complication for an unlimited time. Never, in forty years of treating cancer, have I experienced more positive results than I have with the iridodials. At present, I have begun a research program to biosynthesize iridodials in large quantities, to meet broad clinical demand.

Oncostatins

The genetic structures that cause malignant disorders have been termed the *oncogenes*. Over the last ten years, extensive work has been done in the United States to identify the oncogenes responsible for the cellular disorder we call "cancer." Dr. Todaro, at the National Cancer Institute in

Bethesda, Maryland, has isolated substances from normal genes that are able to reverse the genetic misinformation in cancer cells. These substances are called oncostatins.

In Hannover, Germany, my staff and I are currently using one of these oncostatins—*Ney Tumerin*— to help cancers regress through genetic repair. This approach is especially aimed at the long-term treatment of myelomas and plasma cytomas. But currently, oncostatins are not widely used because they are difficult to produce. Through genetic engineering, we hope to be able to mass-produce them and to figuratively bathe cancer patients in these repair substances to totally erase the cancer's genetic coding.

Squalene (Shark Liver Oil)

Sharks are believed to be millions of years old—actually prehistoric—and are extremely resistant to cancer. Although shark cartilage has been shown to have strong anticancer potential, shark liver oil, containing 60 percent squalene, is many times more effective as a gene-repair and anticancer substance. Furthermore, humans can ingest it readily, without adverse side effects. I have found squalene to be both an effective anticancer and antiviral substance.

Sharks are able to recycle back into the sea the high-sodium concentration that apparently triggers the development of cancer in humans. (Remember, it was previously explained that the profuse amount of sodium in the cancerous cell destroys the electrical condenser function and ultimately disables the cell.) They accomplish this by secreting substances that create an environment of *desodification*, depleting dangerous cells of their sodium and causing them to lose their vitality. Orthodox medical researchers have not pursued studies in desodification, nor is it likely that they will.

Animal studies done in 1996 at Johns Hopkins University School of Medicine report that squalamine—another term for squalene—significantly reduces the growth of new blood vessels feeding solid brain tumors. The tumor's growth is likely to slow down as a result. The head authors of these studies included Allen K. Sills, MD, and Henry Brem, MD, both of Hopkins.

In my opinion, squalene combined with vitamin C (preferably in the form of the ascorbates) is an excellent gene-repair substance. This combination helps the organism develop defense factors against both malignant cells and herpes-type viruses. Squalene and vitamin C also stimulate the body to increase the production of the carcinogen-blocking hormone DHEA and the enzyme cholinesterase. Together with vitamin D (ergocalciferol), these substances assist in the formation of the short-lived tumosterons, which are highly effective anticancer, anti-herpes, genetic-repair substances.

Tumosterons

Another way to correct the cancer cell's genetic misinformation is to use tumosterons, which are repair substances naturally excreted by the lymph cell. They have very short life spans and are quite difficult to isolate experimentally. My staff and I have observed that the tumosterons are ejected from lymph cells that have attached themselves to a tumor cell. Then, by penetrating into the nucleus of that cell, they are able to switch off or reverse the genetic information of malignancy. Here we have an important link between the immuno-defense system—namely, the killer lymph cell coupling with the tumor cell—and the genetic-repair system activated through the production of tumosterons by the lymph cell. The knowledge of this natural genetic repair process helps us to design new strategies for cancer treatment. As mentioned above, the combination of squalene, vitamin C, and vitamin D promote the production of tumosterons in the body.

These gene-repairing and gene-extinguishing substances have become an important part of the broad, nontoxic spectrum of substances that I use to effectively treat my cancer patients and to provide them with a greatly improved quality of life at a fraction of the cost of orthodox cancer therapies. They also point to the fact that extensive and continuing research in the field of genetics is crucial to advance cancer treatment.

GENETICS AND VIRUSES

Genetic instabilities and disease resulting from factors produced in the cellular mitochondria and plasma may be produced when the cell is exposed to radiation; to the intense magnetism of the geopathic zones; or as the result of cellular penetration by specific viruses, such as the cytomegalo, Epstein-Barr, varicella (chickenpox), or herpes viruses. All of these mentioned viruses fall under the general category of herpes simplex. Toxic substances, particularly the sub-components of certain herpes viruses, enter into the mitochondria and may remain there for a very long time. As a matter of fact, I have come to the conclusion that herpes virus interaction within the cellular mitochondria initiates their genetic instability. If we find ways to inactivate or reverse the mitochondrial genetic damage, we have a chance to gain much better control over cancer, for relatively little money.

A dramatic change in our understanding and, subsequently, in our treatment of cancer was witnessed in 1996. With the cooperation of Eva Krompotich, a world-leading authority in herpes virus research who is now working in our Hannover hospital and office, my colleagues and I have discovered the following: There is virtually no malignancy in man that is not associated with elevated cytomegalo, Epstein-Barr, or herpes II virus IGG titers. (IGG titers are the standard diagnostic blood test measurement for determining the presence of herpes and herpes-related viruses).

This discovery means that from less than three months to over three decades before the manifestation of a malignancy, a nucleic component of the cytomegalo/herpes genes (which include about 240,000 base pairs of genes) has entered some of the normal receiving cells of the individual. After possibly years of dormancy within the person's cells, some event may trigger the viral genes to activate, resulting in malignancy, colitis, pulmonary fibrosis, neurodermatitis, rheumatoid diseases, or other chronic diseases.

These findings leave us with a new task: We must try to inactivate the origin of the virus in the cells, to practice prevention. Two antiviral agents, *Retrovir* and *Ganciclovir*, are already used as antivirus treatments, but they are not useful in attacking deep-seated cellular disorder. Retrovir and Ganciclovir are proprietary drugs that are synthesized in laboratories and are considered orthodox treatments. They are active only against the replication of the entire virus, and not against the viral segments that have buried themselves within our cells.

Since 1995, my colleagues and I have been making revolutionary discoveries the could possibly lead to major breakthroughs in cancer therapy. Dr. Davidson, the famous virologist from the University of Chicago, and his long-time associate, Dr. Kropotic from the University of Chicago Medical School, now working with my staff and I in Germany, found that the herpes viruses settle in the B-lymphocytes. It is from the B-lymphocytes that these viruses infect the entire organism with viral sub-components. And these sub-components may lie dormant in the DNA of the cells' mitochondrial membranes for several decades. For some time, we have known that the genetic impulses that instruct the cell nucleus to become malignant come as faulty messages from the infected mitochondrial membranes.

Diseases like colitis, rheumatoid arthritis, pulmonary fibrosis, Lou Gehrig's disease (ALS), and even psoriasis and neurodermatitis seem to follow this same pathogenic pattern. Even the smallest malignant growth is found to be accompanied by a positive test confirming a herpes viral component. This means that in all malignancies, a herpes-type virus has entered and infected the body, ultimately producing the genetic deviation that we know as cancer. If this is true for the other diseases mentioned as well, we are confronted with the insight that viral infection plays a pre-dominant role and may be the common denominator that seems to exist among these illnesses. We are getting closer, at last, to understanding many life-threatening diseases. And after understanding, a cure is not far behind.

I am quite confident that it is possible to bring cancer under control. There are many people who do not get cancer. If we can determine the protective mechanisms that keep these people healthy and then imitate such mechanisms, we can very well defeat cancer. For those who have cancer, follow-ing early diagnosis and immediately following surgery, it is important to start protective therapy for an indefinite peri-od of time. This protective cancer therapy should be based on the use of nontoxic, orthomolecular, gene-repairing sub-stances, as well as sound diet managment.

CHAPTER 8

ᘀNDERSTANDING AND TREATING MULTIPLE SCLEROSIS

Hope for Us! Taking Positive Action Against Multiple Sclerosis . . . .

—Claire V. Morrissette

My original fields of specialization are cancer therapy and the metabolic aspects of the heart, vascular tissue, and skeletal structure. I owe my involvement with multiple sclerosis (MS) to years of scientific and clinical experience as an internist, not as a neurologist. I have an enormous MS practice, having treated over 3,150 ambulatory and non-ambulatory patients from all over the world for this disease over the past thirty years. Eighty percent of my MS patients come from North America.

DEFINING MULTIPLE SCLEROSIS (MS)

Thanks to American research, knowledge about MS has greatly increased in recent years, to the point that it is now possible for me to explain the origin and the fundamentals of this disease. Multiple sclerosis is a progressive, degenerative disease of the central nervous system. It involves destruction of the myelin sheaths around nerve axons, resulting in scar tissue called *plaques* and ultimately destroying the nerves and their ability to function. MS patients experience membrane deterioration. This process is known as *sclerosis*.

In more detail, the *myelin sheath* is a complex membrane layer that is wound around a nerve fiber, referred to as the central axon (see Figure 8.1). The multi-layered sheath is comprised of from five to thirty layers. It resembles a giant tobacco leaf coiled around a central trunk. Each individual layer of the laminated leaf is structurally identical with the membrane of a cell. That means that it has the ability to hold an electrical charge of opposite polarity, thereby functioning as an electrical condenser. It was only recently discovered that this many-layered condenser system acts as an electrical shunt to the central axon.

The myelin sheath, which surrounds the nerve fiber just like insulation around an electric wire, is itself surrounded by the *medullary sheath* or *oligodendroglia,* which is composed of oligodendrocyte cells. These specific cells secrete *myelin*—a lipid or fatty substance that makes up the myelin sheath.

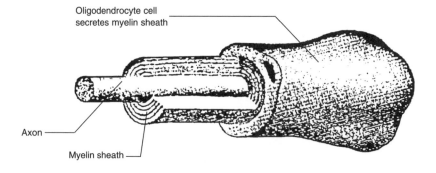

Figure 8.1. The Central Axon and the Myelin Sheath

During MS attacks, the myelin sheath is partially destroyed or demyelated by *killer T-cells*—powerful components of the immune system—leaving patches of scar tissue in the myelin sheath. This scar tissue interrupts communication being sent from the brain and nerve terminals, resulting in various disturbances of the nervous system, such as poor nerve signal transmission, bodily weakness, and similar functional problems.

Symptoms vary among individuals, depending on which portions of the nervous system are most affected. In the early stages, a person may experience episodes of dizziness; emotional mood changes, such as mood swings or depression; eye problems such as blurring or double vision; tingling or numbness, particularly in the extremities; loss of balance or coordination; muscular stiffness; nausea and vomiting; slurred speech; tremors; weakness and fatigue; difficulty in breathing; and in men, impotence. Multiple sclerosis is a general membrane disease, not a nerve cell disease. It is an autoimmune disease that attacks all of the membranes. But the cellular membrane degradation does affect the actual nerve fiber transmission. Many MS patients can't walk and are relegated to wheelchairs. They frequently suffer from degradation of the bones and the organs, such as the adrenals.

MS appears to be more common in temperate climates (1 case per 2,000) than in the tropics (1 case per 100,000), and in large dairy-producing regions of the world. The average onset occurs between the ages of twenty and forty years, and women are more commonly affected than men.

THE MYELIN SHEATH, AEP, AND MEMBRANE INFERIORITY

After many years of studying energy and the body, I have come to believe that the myelin sheath converts vacuum field energy (see pages 25 to 28) into the electrical energy

Blood-Brain-Barrier Type Multiple Sclerosis

A controlled molecular flow of nutrients to the brain is essential for normal brain function. Nutrients enter the brain's blood by passing through capillary walls. Endothelial cells line the capillary walls and are wrapped within fibers of protective neurons (nerve cells), creating an almost impenetrable filter layer, so that harmful substances may be kept out. The relatively small molecules of oxygen, water, and glucose pass easily through this two-layered barrier, but larger molecules, such as those of drugs, toxins, and chemicals, cannot pass to the brain. In some MS patients, we can observe inflammation in this *blood-brain barrier (BBB)*—the simple membrane located between the circulating blood and the brain. This inflammation results in what is called Kowert Type II MS (or BBB Type MS), as opposed to the more common demyelating form of the disease, which is called Kowert Type I MS.

When inflammation of the BBB predominates, a somewhat atypical MS picture arises. An attack of inflammation is accompanied by a migraine-like headache. After becoming extremely severe, the headache finally dissipates. Very often, the diagnosis of BBB Type MS requires a lumbar spinal tap in order to examine the cerebrospinal fluid for evidence of changes that inflammation would cause. I must caution that as little as possible of the fluid should be removed, and once the diagnosis is completed, the procedure should never be repeated. The pressure-stress created by the fluid removal can be most harmful to the BBB, may produce long-lasting headaches, and may cause the disease to worsen. The same is true of X-rays or CAT scans of the brain or spinal cord. By no means should the patient be subjected to repeated taps or any "invasive" diagnostic procedure. Unfortunately, this very important rule is frequently violated.

necessary for the functioning of the central axon. This system can be likened to the automotive Plasma Ignition system now on the market in Germany. Through this Plasma system, the ignition energy of the spark to start the automobile can be strengthened from 100 to 250 times. Considering the number of wrappings (layers) in the myelin sheath, it is possible that the strengthening of the axon energy may be even greater in the human body—more than 100 to 250 times what it otherwise would be—due to this membrane. The sheath acts as a vacuum field energy condenser and amplifier.

There are certain chemical substances necessary for the correct bonding of the electrical charge to the cell membrane of the myelin sheath. One of the most necessary is *aminoethylphosphate*, which is called AEP for short. This substance was first described as an essential component of cell membranes in the 1940s, by the famous American biochemist Dr. Erwin Chargoff. If there is insufficient AEP in the cell membranes, the binding of the electrical charge and the electrical condenser function will be seriously impaired.

My colleagues and I have discovered that in patients with autoimmune disorders, the body does not produce enough AEP to sufficiently supply blood and urine tract cells. Thus, these cells cannot maintain cellular integrity and function. For example, the electrostatic charge of the urinary tract cells is insufficient, and thus the electrostatic defense filter, responsible for keeping the urinary tract clean, does not function adequately. In such cases, there is a constant danger of urinary tract infection. Special credit must be given to American biochemist Galland and to German biochemist Vanselow, both of whom conducted extensive research on this problem. Medical tests indicate the AEP deficiency in the blood and urine not only holds true for those with multiple sclerosis, but also for those who have other immune disorders affecting the lungs, kidneys, and other organs.

During MS attacks, severe polarization of the myelin sheath can be observed. *Polarization* refers to separation of positive and negative electric charges. This leads to the inability of the myelin sheath structure to retain water and to magnetize the structure of the water. Diagnostic magnetic resonance imaging, commonly known as MRI, is able to image and detect MS in the brain. The loss of the nerve cell's condenser function explains why portions of the myelin sheath can be partially destroyed by the killer T-cells of the immune system. When the cellular membrane system is not maintaining proper charges, the membranes lose the ability to defend themselves adequately.

The combination of AEP insufficiency, functional membrane inferiority, and the resulting harm done by immune lymph cells and antibodies leads more or less to total destruction of the myelin through demyelinization disease. This affects and impairs the nerve cells of the spinal column, resulting in loss of muscle control. And remember, it is important to realize that MS attacks all cell membranes, not just those in the myelin sheath. I have observed many side effects in MS patients. For example, the small vascular capillaries become brittle and an assortment of bluish spots appear randomly over the body. In addition, many people with MS experience severe joint pains. When these patients are given the AEP compounds, the brittleness of the capillaries diminishes, the blue spots become fewer, and the individuals even experience less chills.

POSSIBLE CAUSES OF MULTIPLE SCLEROSIS

After many years of working with MS, I have identified several factors that possibly cause the onset of multiple sclerosis. These are: aluminum and other elements; dairy products; geopathic zones; heredity; and viruses.

Aluminum and Other Harmful Elements

Aluminum is strongly suspected of causing damage to membranes and the nervous system. A study of amyotrophic lateral sclerosis (ALS), also known as Lou Gehrig's disease, in Guam revealed a very high incidence of ALS among aluminum welders. I have found evidence of aluminum exposure in my ALS patients as well. ALS is a disease in which brain-stem nerve cells are damaged by components of the herpes virus family, including the cytomegalo, Epstein-Barr, herpes II, and varicella viruses. What does this have to do with MS? There are significant similarities between ALS and MS. The two diseases share similar motor symptoms, such as weakness, problems with walking, and tremors. Both are progressive diseases that can lead to the threatening *medulla oblongata deficiency symptoms*, discussed on page 128. ALS originates with nerve dysfunction; the symptoms of MS result from faulty nerve transmissions that have taken place due to membrane sclerosis. My colleagues and I strongly suspect that aluminum and other harmful elements also play a role in the development of many MS cases. So we are hopeful that the substances that aid in treating ALS can also aid in reducing the symptoms of MS.

I am very suspicious of the influence of aluminum not only in MS and ALS, but also in Alzheimer's disease. It has been established that the brains of people with Alzheimer's have ten to thirty times as much aluminum as the normal brain. We are exposed to aluminum constantly, in pots and pans, through aluminum hydroxide in many deodorants, and in U.S. soda-pop cans. It is best to avoid the ingestion and use of products encased in or exposed to this element.

In addition to the detrimental effects of aluminum, there are other elements that are known to harm cell membranes and the nervous system. Some of these are: fluorine; platinum; nickel; mercury and silver (amalgam fillings in the teeth); chromium; and other heavy metals. These substances are poisonous and, by nature, destructive to the electrical function of the cell membrane.

Dairy Products

MS is most prevalent in dairy-producing regions worldwide. There are two theories that explain the close relationship between dairy consumption and MS. The first one assumes that there are virus particles in milk that act as "starter viruses" and bring about the disease. The other theory originated and was researched in England about thirty years ago. It involves *glutens,* immune-active sugar-albumin complexes found in milk (and possibly in cereals), which can also activate the condition so that it becomes clinically evident.

Heredity

There appears to be some inherited predisposition to the body's inability to supply adequate amounts of AEP to the cellular membranes. As discussed earlier in this chapter, sufficient AEP is necessary to bind the proper electrical charge of the cell membrane. Incorrect membrane charge can lead to multiple sclerosis, among many other disorders. I have particularly noted this apparent familial multiple sclerosis defect exhibited in mother and child and in identical twins.

Geopathic Zones

A major factor associated with the manifestation of MS is the effect of geopathic zones (see page 126), which will cause imbalance in the proper electrostatic recharging of the membrane. In 1984, I treated an MS patient who lived in northern California. Her husband reported that they lived in a region of continual earthquake activity and not far from a place where a person must stand at an angle to keep from falling down. In this region, the incidence of MS is greater than 4,000 per million—more than ten times the average incidence across the country! Such an observation stresses that the effects of geopathic zones must not be ignored, and that individuals with multiple sclerosis should be removed from these zones.

Viruses

In order to understand the onset of MS, we need to know the underlying cause of immune aggression that works against the myelin. There is no doubt in my mind that this autoimmune process is initiated by a viral infection. Initially, it starts out as a healing action to destroy bacteria and other foreign protein invaders, but later, it somehow develops properties of its own, which, after a latency period, become programmed not only to destroy the initial virus, but also to attack the myelin membrane structure (perhaps the oligodendroglia that forms the myelin) and occasionally the blood-brain-barrier (see page 118).

There are numerous viruses suspected. The most significant virus seems to be measles. This was revealed by Dr. Mannweiler, a Hamburg (Germany) neurologist who has stated, "Everyone, every patient with MS—and I mean 100 percent—had a severe bout with measles, or has been exposed to a measles-type virus."

A significant number of Americans became sick with MS in 1978. A very high percentage of these had swine flu immunization in 1977. Another equally important starter virus is thought to be canine distemper. Additional suspected viruses are those of the mumps, chickenpox (the varicella virus), and possibly smaller virus segments.

ORTHODOX THERAPIES FOR MS

Several decades ago, a *smear cure of a mercury salve* was recommended in an attempt to block the autoimmune MS process. Some positive clinical effects were reported, but the prevalent side effect of kidney damage was extensive. Therefore, this therapy is no longer suggested.

A medication recommended today for its immune-inhibiting ability is *azathioprine* (Imuran, Imurex). I believe it is essential to warn patients that azathioprine will cause liver damage if used for any length of time. In addition, there is an increased susceptibility to viral infection and possibly even cancer. The toxic effects of this therapy must be carefully considered.

Then there is *cyclophosphamide* (Cytoxan, Endoxan). Occasionally, American doctors prescribe this in highly toxic doses, and we see these patients with their hair falling out and with severe bone-marrow damage. For this reason, I think it is not advisable to use this substance. There is a much better alternative—the chemically related *trophosphamide* (Ixoten). This is just as effective as other immunosuppressive substances, and it is tolerated far better over a longer period of time. My staff and I have used Ixoten for about twenty years now, at low dose levels for ten to twelve weeks. Even Ixoten therapy is truly only useful for a limited period of time, albeit a longer period than those of the other medications.

Prescribing *ACTH* (adrenocorticotropic hormone) to MS patients has become a widespread habit—or perhaps I should say, a widespread bad habit. ACTH stimulates the adrenal cortex to secrete minerals and glucocorticoids which, in turn, control chemical constitution of body fluids, metabolism, and secondary sexual characteristics. While there is often temporary improvement, the long-run result of ACTH use is one of steady deterioration. If ACTH is to be given for a short time, it is absolutely necessary to supply the foods required of the adrenal cortex systems—raw foods, vitamin D_2, vitamin C (in large doses), beta-carotene, and especially selenium. I should emphasize that I have not used ACTH at all for the past twenty years.

MY MS TREATMENT PROGRAM

Taking into account the extensive experience I have had in treating MS, I have created the following program for the individual with multiple sclerosis. It involves a commitment to healthy lifestyle habits—good diet, regular exercise, and a clean environment—and to the regular use of alternative orthomolecular substances.

Diet, Exercise, and Environment

I must stress the extreme importance of a good diet. I recommend avoiding milk and milk products as far as possible. An exception is allowed for natural French cheese, in which the glutens have been broken down by fermentation. A strict diet of raw, organically grown foods is best. When cooking and eating, avoid using aluminum cookware or beverages stored in aluminum cans.

In addition to this dietary advice, I recommend controlled exercise and plenty of rest. Both active and passive (secondary) smoking are strictly forbidden. The so-called *nicotine* or *cotinine effect* is mainly brought about by an impairment of the electrical properties of the cell membrane. This was discovered by Henri Laborit, French scientist and my friend of many years. Any exposure to this poisonous smoke should be avoided. It is also essential to

avoid fluorinated water, fluorinated toothpaste, and fluorinated mouthwash. Chlorinated water may also be harmful. Another suggested and important safety measure is to
have all silver-mercury amalgam fillings in your teeth
replaced with composition.

It must be determined if you live or spend much time in a
geopathic zone. This can be done using a geo-magnetometer,
such as the Meersman device, but a well-qualified dowser (a
person trained in the use of a divining rod to find water) is
the best person to turn to for this determination. If it is found
that you are in a geopathic zone, consider moving to another region in the same house—one that is free of this destructive geopathic energy. Usually, the geopathic energy is highly specific to one area; it is often confined, for example, to one
room. A heavy duty copper wire installed around the complete foundation of the house and grounded to a copper pipe
will usually "bleed off" the geopathic energy.

Alternative Substances

The most important part of my treatment for MS is an
attempt to correct the chemical and electrical defects of the
cell membrane. The remedies of choice are the 2-AEP salts
or colamine phosphate salts, including calcium 2-AEP and
the 2-AEP complex (see pages 62 to 67). You may recall
from earlier discussions in this text that these were synthesized for me by the late Dr. Franz Kohler in Germany. The
project was carried out with the intent to find a highly
effective membrane-sealing substance to protect against
the intrusion of viruses, bacteria, and toxic antibodies. The
ability of substances such as calcium 2-AEP to bind an electrical charge on the myelin sheath membrane is a special
physiological quality. Such substances are called *neurotransmitters.* Also, because calcium aspartate (see page 56)
produces a similar effect, my staff and I have added it to
our protocol as an anti-immunological sealing substance.

Some of our patients have been successfully treated solely with calcium aspartate for over thirty years.

In 1968, the German Health Authority (the Bundesgesundheitampt—the equivalent of the American FDA) declared calcium 2-AEP an official medication in the treatment of multiple sclerosis. In 1986, Dr. George N. Morrisette in the United States conducted an extensive retrospective study on the effect of calcium 2-AEP on over 250 American MS patients. His findings reveal that a positive response rate of about 80 percent supported my MS clinical results in Germany.

At Hannover, my colleagues and I discovered that both the 2-AEP salts and the aspartates function as neurotransmitters and are needed for the binding and flow of the electrical charge on the cell membrane. We give our patients daily tablets of both the 2–AEP complex and calcium 2-AEP. Part of the calcium 2-AEP must be administered by IV-injection, as this is the only way to initially build a sufficient concentration of the calcium phosphate on the cell membrane. An interruption of this IV therapy almost inevitably results in a definite worsening of the disease. The combined therapy should be continued for an unlimited time. In select cases, the IV-injection method can be replaced by a much higher oral intake of calcium 2-AEP or the 2-AEP complex.

It is important to note that whether a patient is taking calcium aspartate or the 2-AEP complex, the oral intake must be continued for the individual's entire life. The metabolic bodily processes of a person afflicted with MS indicate the production of AEP will be impaired for life. Thus, any current or former MS patient must remain on the therapeutic substances even after a positive effect has been experienced, so that the cell membranes remain properly functional.

In addition, I give my patients calcium orotate—the mineral salt of orotic acid. (Orotic acid is also known as vitamin

B$_{13}$.) Calcium orotate produces a sealing effect on the surface of the membranes of intracellular structures like the mitochondria. It also favorably influences the inflammation of the blood-brain barrier and the inner structure of the oligodendroglia cells. The calcium orotate therapy is increased for MS patients displaying migraine-like headaches that almost always disappear. This is also true of lithium orotate, the most effective medication I have found for the treatment of migraines. It is very helpful in the treatment of Type Kowert II MS. (See "Blood-Brain-Barrier Type Multiple Sclerosis," page 118. Also, for further information on the orotates, see pages 58 to 60.)

My staff and I have introduced squalene, with ascorbates, to our MS patients, and we have gotten promising results. Squalene is shark liver oil tripertenoid a very old biogenetic mother-substance of steroids and other components that perform the immune surveillance function. (See page 109 for more inforamtion on squalene.) Patients treated with squalene report feeling warmer, particularly in their extremities, no longer experienceing the characteristic MS chills.

I must give special consideration to the propensity of the individual with MS to develop infections of the urinary tract. For long-term protection, we use a sulfonamide called Harnosal. It is not so much the bactericidal function of the sulfonamide that is effective, but the electrostatic activity that the Harnosal restores to the urinary passage cells.

SUCCESSFUL RESULTS

The rate of success following our treatments and therapies varies. As a rule, the response in patients with early-onset, shorter-term illness is much greater than in patients with advanced illness. I have found that Americans respond much better to my treatment regimen than to any of the other conventional treatments that their healthcare system offers. Generally, my therapy results in fairly reliable improvement—at least partly back to normal—of the bladder function, the intestinal sphincter muscles, and voluntary control of the big toe, even with badly crippled patients. In addition, the upper body functions are also improved, lessening the following: vertigo; slurred speech; loss of facial expression control; loss of motor function of the arm and hand; and especially the *medulla oblongata deficiency symptoms*. This last group of very dangerous symptoms includes the inability to swallow, defective breathing functions, and poor regulation of circulation. These symptoms also occur with ALS and may be handled with continuous protection offered by the mineral salts of colamine phosphate (2-AEP), as well.

Unfortunately, the disturbed motor function of the upper thigh muscles, those essential to walking, are quite resistant to my therapy, or at least improvement has been noted in only a few. This can be avoided if therapy is started early. Over the course of more than five years, of 100 patients who started therapy while still ambulatory, only two have been reduced to using a wheelchair. Normally, about one-quarter of all MS patients eventually die of extreme bone degeneration and fractures. I have observed only eight bone fractures among over 3,150 MS patients treated with calcium 2-AEP over a thirty-year period. Furthermore, a group of MS patients who I first saw and treated in 1968 have not experienced any further progression of their disease and continue to follow my strict treatment and advice.

In 1987, the Keith Brewer Foundation and Science Library presented the 4th Annual New Horizons in Health Seminar. Both Drs. Franz Kohler and George N. Morrisette gave brilliant lectures on my calcium 2-AEP as a leading therapy for multiple sclerosis. The audience's reaction was very positive; there was an immediate outcry and demand that the U.S. FDA make this therapy readily available to

MS patients throughout the country. It is important to understand that calcium 2-AEP powders, administered in capsules/tablets, are approved for use in the United States, but the more powerful intravenous (IV) therapy is not. It was this IV treatment to which Americans want and deserve access. There are hundreds of individuals with MS who, each year and every day, are suffering and dying because they cannot freely access this nontoxic therapy. One is forced to ask: What has happened to freedom of choice in the Land of the Free and the Brave?

CHAPTER 9

*F*AME AND INFAMY

Men cling to the opinions to which they are accustomed,
this prevents them from finding the truth.

—Moses Maimonides (1135–1204)

A s a researcher and clinician at the cutting edge of medical science, I have received a lot of attention. At times,
the spotlight has been helpful, for increased exposure means
that more people can gain hope and health through my
work. I have made many friends and have received much
support. But that same spotlight has also been the source of
much defamation, as advocates and members of conventional medicine and the pharmaceutical industry react negatively, sometimes out of fear and at other times out of greed.

THE START OF SOMETHING BIG

During the late 1960s and early 1970s, several world-class scientists and humanitarians from North America influenced

my thinking and early work in the development of non-toxic substances that effectively prevent and treat cancer. These great men were: Dr. Ernst T. Krebs, Jr.; Dr. Dean Burk; Andrew R.L. McNaughton; and Dr. Linus Pauling. Through my association and correspondence with them over the years, many Americans, including some of the rich and famous, have learned that I offer viable therapeutic alternatives to the American medical establishment's conventional therapies.

Biochemist Dr. Ernst T. Krebs, Jr.—son of the late Dr. Ernst Krebs, MD, of San Francisco, who discovered and used Laetrile—carried on his father's work despite extreme government harassment and persecution. Throughout years of conflict, Dr. Krebs, Jr., maintained a close alliance with Andrew R.L. McNaughton, founder and president of the McNaughton Foundation, a primary sponsor of Laetrile research around the world. In his book *Vitamin B$_{17}$—Forbidden Weapon Against Cancer*, Michael Culbert discusses the McNaughton Foundation, which started in 1956. He explains its purpose of sponsoring research that promises breakthroughs in important new areas where sufficient professional acceptance (and funding) does not exist. The McNaughton Foundation also aims to sponsor the very best scientist for the specific job in his own research institution, wherever it may be in the world. Finally, this foundation focuses upon transforming into reality new solutions to the problems of mankind.

I initially learned about Laetrile (amygdalin) at the 1966 International Cancer Congress in Tokyo. After suitable testing had been done on the substance, I began using amygdalin on my cancer patients with some success. Andrew McNaughton first consulted with me in Germany in 1970, inquiring about the results obtained from my clinical use of amygdalin and the chemical mandelonitriles. He subsequently asked me to become a member of his foundation's advisory board. I did, joining other prominent members of

Andrew R.L. McNaughton

Andrew R.L. McNaughton is the son of the late General A.G.L. McNaughton, commander of the Canadian Armed Forces in World War II and a former President of the United Nations Security Council and the Canadian National Research Council. Andrew graduated with an arts degree from Loyola College in Montreal, and gained additional degrees in electrical engineering at the Royal Military College in Kingston, Ontario; in geology and mining at McGill University in Montreal; and in business administration at the Alexander Hamilton Institute. During World War II, Andrew was awarded the Air Force Cross for his work as the chief test pilot and commander of the Royal Canadian Air Force's Experimental Test and Development Center. His many scientific associations include membership in the New York Academy of Sciences and the Royal Society of Medicine.

the board, including Dr. Ernst T. Krebs, Jr.; Dr. Manfred von Ardenne, President of the Manfred von Ardenne Research Institute of Dresden, Germany; Dr. Fedor Trimus, Professor of Pharmacology in the Ukrainian Ministry of Public Health in Kyiv, Ukraine; and Dr. Dean Burke of the National Cancer Institute.

It was Dr. Ernst Krebs, Jr., who initially told Andrew McNaughton about Alicia Button's terminal cancer, and how her physicians had given her only six months to live. McNaughton convinced Alicia and her husband, the great actor and comedian Red Buttons, to consult with me in 1972. My success in treating Alicia's cancer became widespread knowledge in Hollywood and brought me considerable recognition, for my therapy was credited with saving her life. An example of the attention that I began to receive through the media can be found in the following excerpt that appeared in the February 20, 1980 edition of the *Hollywood Reporter.* The article, titled "The Great Life," was written by columnist George Christy.

> Dr. Hans Nieper, the German genius who has cured Alecia Buttons, Fred MacMurray and art dealer Chuck Feingarten of cancer, stopped in Los Angeles for several days, and his first evening was with his favorite booster, Edie Goetz (daughter of the late movie mogul, Louis B. Mayer), who invited Dr. Nieper's "cures" and friends to one of her glorious buffet dinners. . . . Nieper's wife, Helga, accompanied him on this visit, where he is exploring "gravity research" theories . . . .

The article went on to mention additional celebrity personalities who were interested in and/or involved with my work, including Natalie Wood and Robert Wagner. Thus, I was getting high-profile media exposure regarding my alternative cancer therapies.

I returned to Germany that spring, after a successful speaking tour in the United States. However, the spotlight on my alternative cancer treatments remained hot. Congressman Larry McDonald of Georgia, Sponsor of the *H.R. 4045* bill to legalize the use of Laetrile, addressed Congress on March 31, 1980. He explained that Laetrile was successfully being used as a standard treatment in other countries, including Germany, and informed the House of Representatives of the widespread support for my work with this substance. Then McDonald commended to his colleagues several of my statements from a Gertrude Engels Public Relations Firm press release dated March 15, 1980, including my opinion that the FDA was creating trouble that was not found elsewhere in the world. One of my statements that was read to the House of Representatives was the following: "I cannot believe it. What is the stir of the Food and Drug Administration 'Grandfather clause' to determine the validity of Laetrile when we have had success all over the world? We don't have this trouble in Germany."

THE HEAVY HAND OF THE FDA

As my visibility as a physician and spokesman for alternative, orthomolecular medicine grew throughout the United States, so did the resentment from the orthodox medical establishment. I quickly became a primary target of the watchdogs of the FDA, who branded me that "infamous" German doctor who is promoting "unproven, illegal drugs." The FDA set their regulatory procedures into motion, publishing Import Alerts on shipments of the vital medications, vitamins, and minerals that I had prescribed for my American patients during their treatment at my clinic in Germany. These FDA Import Alerts instructed its agents and U.S. Customs personnel to enforce "Automatic Detention of 'Unapproved' New Drugs Promoted by Dr. Hans Nieper of Germany."

"Unapproved" does not mean that a drug doesn't work, but merely that the new drug or medication has not been tested under the rigid FDA requirements for safety and efficacy. Among these tests are the very costly *double-blind evaluations*, which require administering the test substance to one group of patients while giving a placebo—an inert or inactive substance—to another group (known as the control group) for objective evaluation of the substance. I can understand why these controls were instituted in 1962, following the thalidomide disaster. Thalidomide was a widely prescribed sedative that was found to cause terrible birth defects in the children of pregnant women who took the substance. This "approved" drug had to be pulled off the market. After such a horrendous situation, the FDA set heavy standards for drugs to be extensively tested before being approved. So it is understandable why the FDA has established tight requirements when it comes to dealing with new synthetic, toximolecular medications. However, many vitamin, mineral, herbal, and other natural supplements are *not* prescription drugs and should *not* be classified and treated as such. Yet the FDA clearly wanted to gain control over all of the substances that I prescribed, which, incidentally, are available over-the-counter in all of the European countries, Mexico, and Asia.

The following extract is part of an Import Alert that was published in late 1985 and broadly distributed by the FDA. It attempted to vilify and discredit me as a physician and to deny my American patients access to vitally needed, legally licensed medications prescribed by me during their therapy in Germany.

Hans A. Nieper, a West German physician, has claimed for some years to have treatments for cancer, heart disease and multiple sclerosis. He utilizes a mix of numerous minerals, vitamins and animal and plant extracts for which therapeutic representations are made, and other drugs, for which he has not sought U.S. approval. Dr. Nieper travels in the United States on speaking engagements which encourage patients to go to Germany for his unorthodox "treatments."

Since September 1985, FDA has issued notices and advised bringing these products into the United States in their baggage or receiving them by mail that, contrary to what they may have been led to believe, these unapproved products are illegal and may be detained in the future. Almost always, the drugs are labeled in German with no English-language labeling, and seldom do they contain directions for use. FDA has advised Dr. Nieper and shippers of these products from West Germany regarding the illegali-

ty of these shipments and has told them of the need to provide scientific data and otherwise follow U.S. procedures
designed to protect U.S. citizens (and U.S. Pharmaceutical
Companies) from unproven, unsafe and ineffective products. Despite this advice, shipments of these unapproved
products have continued.

Dr. Nieper has taken no steps to bring the products into
compliance. As a result, FDA is now working with the U.S.
Customs Service to halt this illegal flow. FDA regrets the
impact that may be felt by patients who were misled into
believing the drugs could be legally imported.

There is no requirement for me, a licensed medical doctor practicing in Germany, to obtain FDA approvals on any
of the substances and medications I successfully use in my
practice. I frequently stressed that the medications prescribed by me in Germany are officially licensed by the
German Federal Health Authority and meet accepted
world standards. Responsibility for seeking FDA approvals
for new drugs and medications lies with the prospective
drug manufacturers. Furthermore, there presently isn't, nor
should there ever be, any restriction on my accepting invi-
tations to speak in the United States (or anyplace else in the
world, for that matter). Naturally, many Americans attended my lectures because they were searching for different
(perhaps more promising) avenues of treatment for cancer,
multiple sclerosis, heart disease, and other chronic illnesses.
And many found hope in what they heard. Because alternative therapies were either not available or virtually out-
lawed in the United States, many individuals subsequently
came to me for treatment in Germany.

As the FDA harassment intensified, many critically ill
cancer patients returning home from my clinic in Germany
were detained by U.S. Customs agents on FDA orders.
Their prescribed nontoxic medications, minerals, and nutritional supplements were seized, and my patients were

made to feel like criminals. Thus, they were stripped of their essential medical supplies, stripped of their dignity and freedom of choice, and most importantly, stripped of their chances for survival. These interruptions of therapy led to the premature deaths of many of my cancer patients who may have survived, or at least many who may have had the opportunity to live a few more relatively comfortable years not subject to the conventional radiation and toxic chemotherapy treatments that had failed them. This was how the FDA "protected" American citizens from my therapeutic treatments.

Of course, I was appalled by the false accusations levied against me by the FDA. I vehemently protested the interception of the medications routinely sent to my American patients, but to no avail. On June 17, 1986, I wrote to Senator William Proxmire, whom I had met on several occasions, concerning a letter he had written in response to a constituent's frustration over the FDA's ban on my medications. I took the liberty of telling the Senator that his letter, based undoubtedly on information provided him by the FDA, contained a number of highly incorrect and misleading statements. I assured him that I do not "promote" drugs in the United States and have never done so. I live and work in the Federal Republic of Germany, where I head the medical department of an officially licensed hospital at which I conduct my practice. We are specialized in the treatment of malignancies and immuno-diseases including multiple sclerosis. We routinely see patients from over sixty-seven countries. I informed him that I am not the "proprietor" of the clinic as the FDA claimed, but rather that it belongs to the Paracelsus Hospital Corporation.

I pointed out that the medications I prescribe are not "my drugs," but are manufactured by German companies and are officially licensed by the government, some for over twenty years. In addition, I stated that it is not my concern to ask for the licensing of German medications in

The Kefauver Amendment Changes the Health Industry

Thalidomide, a legal prescription drug, was found to cause severe birth defects in children whose mothers took it while pregnant. In response, President Kennedy, in August of 1962, sent a "consumer-protection" measure to Congress, requesting better federal controls over the sale of dangerous drugs, stronger controls over barbiturates and amphetamines, and the institution of a pre-market testing approach to cosmetics.

Next, Senator Estes Kefauver introduced *Senate bill S1552* in response to the thalidomide scare. This bill: (1) Authorized the FDA to set standards for good manufacturing practices to assure that drugs were produced properly; (2) Required the manufacturer of a substance to demonstrate to the FDA that it was effective, as well as safe, before it could be approved as a "new drug" and marketed; (3) In the case of a previously approved "new drug," in order to determine if its application should be withdrawn on safety grounds, the burden of proof was on the manufacturer to demonstrate that the drug was safe and should be left on the market; (4) Permitted the Secretary of Health, Education and Welfare (HEW) to prohibit further sale of a previously approved "new drug," with a hearing later, if he thought the drug presented an imminent danger to the public safety; (5) Abolished the rule under which, if a "new drug" application was not rejected by the FDA within 60 to 180 days, the application was automatically considered approved. Under this new law, no "new drug" application could be granted without positive FDA approval. There were nine additional powers granted to the FDA under this bill, which gave them almost total control over the preclinical and clinical testing, production, labeling, and marketing of any new drug.

The Kefauver bill was passed by a "78 to 0" roll call vote of the Senate on August 23, 1962. Prior to the Kefauver bill, the burden of proof for efficacy and safety on any new drug rested on the FDA. Now it rests on the research institute that promotes it.

foreign countries. Furthermore, I explained that some of our officially licensed German health products, such as calcium 2-aminoethylphosphate (calcium 2-AEP), were developed under U.S. government funding, and that calcium 2-AEP is by far the most effective long-term treatment for multiple sclerosis. I informed the Senator that cancer patients in Germany have been treated successfully with so-called gene-repair agents, as well. Thus, I stressed the importance of allowing American citizens the freedom of choice to select the substances that I use in my clinic.

The truth is that ever since the adoption of the Kefauver Amendment in 1960 to 1961, the United States has been falling behind in the treatment of chronic diseases. (See "The Kefauver Amendment Changes the Health Industry," page 139.) More and more U.S. citizens are forced to go to foreign countries to find alternative therapies. Unfortunately, only those with money can afford to do so.

THE HARMFUL POLITICS OF RESEARCH AND HEALTHCARE

The American Cancer Society (ACS) has provided research grant-funding to many research institutes for the testing and development of new anticancer agents. From the 1950s through President Nixon's unsuccessful "War on Cancer" in the 1970s, large pharmaceutical companies and university laboratories were encouraged to submit new proprietary chemical substances for confidential testing by such key research institutes as Sloan-Kettering Institute in New York City; Southern Research Institute of Birmingham; the Children's Cancer Research Foundation in Boston; Roswell Memorial Park in Buffalo; and others.

Let's look at an example of the way the ACS, research facilities, and the pharmaceutical industry are tied to one another. One of the most powerful toxic anticancer agents discovered during testing at Sloan-Kettering Institute is 5-Fluorouracil (5-FU). Since 5-FU was tested under an ACS screening grant, the ACS has derived a 50-percent royalty on every gram of 5-FU used in therapy. It is easy to understand why the ACS works so closely with its pharmaceutical industry overlords. To ensure continuity in this cooperative relationship and to protect its vested interests in the "multi-billion dollar a year" cancer industry, many of the key executives and professional staff of the ACS rotate to and from the pharmaceutical industry and the leading cancer research institutes and laboratories.

As Ralph Moss describes in his excellent book *Questioning Chemotherapy*, the ACS fundraising is based on hope and fear. Moss explains that, by provoking a "cancer-phobia" in the general public and then releasing news of a promising drug therapy, the ACS collects millions of dollars in donations. Many hopeful contributors wait with baited breath, only to be disappointed as time passes and no "cure" is found. Also keep in mind that, years ago, the ACS refused to endorse or acknowledge the value of vitamin C and other antioxidants, such as beta-carotene and vitamin E, as cancer preventives. Today, the ACS sells its product endorsement of Florida orange juice as a cancer preventive.

The FDA is a captive of the giant pharmaceutical industry that it proports to regulate. Quite simply, its restrictions and regulations slow things down and keep medicine rather static for long periods of time. Thus, the pharmaceutical giants can reap more money for longer periods of time. The process of finding new substances to treat ill people has been reduced, above all else, to a monetary issue. And alternative medicine, as a field, does not have the money to win the fight.

From about 1986 to 1994, the situation worsened. American physicians were prosecuted, fined, and their licenses to practice medicine stripped away by a bureaucratic coalition of the American Medical Association, the State Boards of Health, the National Cancer Institute, and the FDA, for using "unapproved" nutrient supplements, vitamins, etc. in the treatment of life-threatening diseases. In 1993, Federal search warrants were issued and numerous raids were conducted by Federal agents against American manufacturers of many of the vitamins, minerals, and other supplements that I prescribe for my American patients. These manufacturers' finished products, raw material inventories, records, and even their computers were confiscated. In several cases, the corporate principals were arrested. It was hard for me to imagine that this could happen in a "free" society like that of the United States!

It became obvious to me and to many other health professionals committed to the practice of effective orthomolecular alternative therapies, that the FDA, the American Medical Association, the State Medical Boards of Health, the American Cancer Society, and the National Cancer Institute were doing everything in their power to restrict U.S. patients from the freedom of access to effective alternative cancer therapies. And such therapies are available in many countries outside the United States. The United States Constitution and Bill of Rights guarantee U.S. citizens many freedoms, but apparently not the freedom of choice in health-related matters.

Frequently, governmental regulatory agencies become captive to the very industries they are initially mandated to regulate. In this case, the FDA became subject to the force of the powerful U.S. pharmaceutical industry. The production, sale, and distribution of "officially" approved proprietary cancer drugs contributes to the $12 billion-a-year cancer industry, which constitutes a legalized monopoly. This, of course, is immediately threatened by the introduction of any "unapproved," low-cost, nontoxic cancer therapy.

THE EFFORTS AND SUCCESSES OF ALTERNATIVE THERAPY PROPONENTS

Many grassroots organizations were formed in the United States to challenge the unreasoning power of the FDA. These groups included health professionals; manufacturers and distributors of vitamins, minerals, and health-related medical products and equipment; and publishers of medical books and journals on alternative health care and complementary approaches (those that work in conjunction with conventional therapies). Many of these organizations, including the Cancer Control Society, The International Association for Cancer Victims and Friends, and other self-help organizations too numerous to mention, have worked diligently for over thirty years to bring about greater patient freedom of choice in alternative and complementary cancer therapies. Three organizations have been particularly effective in bringing these issues to the public's attention and before the U.S. Congress in recent years: Citizens for Health; the National Health Freedom Foundation; and the Foundation for the Advancement of Innovative Medicine.

Citizens for Health, founded in Washington State in 1991, has been very effective in sponsoring and promoting legislation focused on restoring freedom of health choices to the American people. Their efforts aim at limiting the power of the FDA to regulate and control alternative therapies and nutritional supplements, which the FDA has labeled "drugs."

The National Health Foundation is committed to working "to ensure a health care system in which health practitioners can practice in conscience with the well being of the patient foremost in their minds without fear of recrimination." This organization helps and defends practitioners of alternative therapies, such as holistic and homeopathic medicine, herbalists, acupuncturists, and naturopaths.

The Foundation for the Advancement of Innovative Medicine (FAIM) was founded in 1989 as a voice for innovative medicine's professionals, patients, and suppliers. This foundation defines innovative medicine as a treatment or therapy of empirical clinical benefit that is yet outside the mainstream of conventional medicine. Innovative medicine is complementary to conventional medicine, offering alternatives as an individual situation may warrant. FAIM's goals are: the development of a membership to serve as both a forum for exchange and a constituency for change; to educate both those within the field and the general public, as to the benefits and issues of innovative medicine; and to secure freedom of choice and guaranteed reimbursement for the patients, be it through legislation, litigation, or negotiation with state agencies and insurance companies. Lastly, in laying the groundwork for a climate receptive to medical innovation, FAIM encourages the research and development of promising new approaches.

In 1992, I was invited to the regulatory offices of the U.S. FDA, under the direction of Deputy Commissioner Albert Rothschild. There, I met with six or seven FDA officials who, with only one exception, were kind and considerate people. The spouse of one of these officials had just been diagnosed with ovarian cancer, and my help was requested. They quickly stated, "Well, the problems you have encountered are not with us, they are with the 'law.'" I responded that they should change the law for the benefit of deserving people. As one body, they took a deep breath.

Over a period of a year and a half, the situation changed entirely. We have reached agreement that every U.S. patient returning from my clinic in Germany will be entitled to keep and receive medications prescribed for his or her disease, provided that the patient's local doctor or medical specialist confirm this disease. In fact, one lady wrote to me that her doctors at the Mayo Clinic and the National Institutes of Health had recommended she consult with me! I therefore ask my American readers to have confidence in the majority of FDA officials. Times change rapidly, and we change with these.

In 1993, as a direct result of the successful lobbying by the above-discussed groups and because of the great public outcry over U.S. restrictions placed on alternative therapies readily available offshore, the Office of Alternative Medicine (OAM) was established by Congress within the National Institutes of Health. This was the first step towards the recognition and acceptance of alternative medicine and its practitioners. The OAM had an initial budget of $2 million; in fiscal 1999, that budget was raised to $50 million.

Shortly after establishing this Office, the United States Congress also passed the Dietary Supplement Health and Education Act of 1994 (DSHEA), which brought relief to the manufacturers and distributors of dietary supplements by allowing them to make limited nutritional support statements about their products without fear of FDA retaliation. And finally, my American patients are once again allowed to bring in, and to receive by mail, essential medications I legally prescribe for them in Germany.

However, the FDA will not allow many of these medications and nutrient supplements to be manufactured and sold in the United States without extensive preclinical and clinical trials to determine if they meet FDA standards of efficacy and safety. The cost of just one of these tests may exceed tens of millions of dollars, a restrictive amount for a small company to pay to gain FDA approval. Thus, the FDA continues to retain much of its ability to protect the proprietary position of the major drug and pharmaceutical companies from competition by the so-called "unapproved, illegal" alternative drugs and substances.

In 1997, several other important legislative bills were introduced in the House of Representatives by Congressman Peter DeFazio, as a result of effective citizen action demanding greater freedom of choice in health care and a curtailment of the FDA's control over alternative and complementary medicine. House bills *H.R. 746*, "To allow patients to receive any medical treatment they want under certain conditions," and *H.R. 1055*, "To establish within the National Institutes of Health an agency to be known as the National Center for Integral Medicine, and for other purposes," are positive indications of the power and effectiveness of citizen action. These bills are fighting to restore and preserve every patient's access to alternative therapies and modalities, as well as to restore the right of the practitioner to practice medicine according to his oath and conscience, without fear of bureaucratic retribution.

Having traveled and lectured in many countries throughout the world, I find it both sad and curious that only in the United States is a physician not free to practice medicine according to his or her knowledge and training. The physician may actually be sued, have his or her license stripped, or even be imprisoned for using every reasonable medication or therapy (including those offered by alternative and complementary medicine) known to him or her and considered of value in the prevention and treatment of disease. I hope the United States government will soon recognize the value of alternative medical modalities, which are available throughout the rest of the world, and that it will provide its citizens with unrestricted access to the latest and best healthcare modalities available by including these alternative medicines as complementary healthcare measures to orthodox medicine. The time has come!

CHAPTER 10

A MORE REASONED APPROACH

The responsibility for the well being of an individual's own body must be returned to the individual.

—Hans A. Nieper, MD (b. 1928)

With the passage of time and the inability of orthodox medicine to tackle the problems of heart disease, cancer, multiple sclerosis, etc., it is becoming increasingly apparent that alternative medicine is the medicine of the future. The greatest minds in medical research and clinical practice have come to this conclusion. Medical progress has continued throughout the centuries because brave pioneers of medicine have convinced the general population that change is good. Let us hope that the politics of health care do not bring this trend of advancement to a halt. Let us hope that an unwavering loyalty to convention and its short-term benefits does not limit the treatment options of people who are suffering from disease.

DR. LINUS PAULING'S PREDICTIONS

As I look with hope to the future, I am reminded of a very important meeting I attended in the spring of 1974. The International Academy of Preventive Medicine invited me to speak about my research and clinical work on mineral transport substances at a congress held at the Hilton Hotel in Washington, D.C. This conference proved to be a landmark event and profoundly influenced my future career. Among the distinguished speakers who delivered brilliant lectures were Nobel Laureate Dr. Linus Pauling, who coined the term *orthomolecular;* Dr. Hans Selye, a Montreal physician who demonstrated that magnesium chloride could protect experimental animal hearts from chemically induced tissue degeneration; Roger Williams, the high priest of vitamin therapy from Austin, Texas; Dr. Ben Cohen, the renowned specialist in diabetes, from Jerusalem; Dr. Bob McCullough, a well-known orthopedic surgeon and Lions International President; and Carlton Fredericks, the most respected disciple of Casimir Funk. (Funk coined the term *vitamin* in 1922.)

At a party following the conference, Dr. Dean Burk, a former division director of the National Cancer Institute, seated me next to Dr. Linus Pauling. During our conversation that evening, Linus shared some of his innermost convictions on the practice of medicine. I remember his words as follows:

> Hans, I believe that substances presently used in the prevention and treatment of chronic diseases that are not orthomolecular [natural substances that restore functional balance to cells and biological systems] will fail. Over the long term, our bodies will simply refuse to respond to treatment with nonorthomolecular substances. Orthodox medicine will attempt to compensate for its disregard of this maxim, [a disregard] which is born of narrow-mindedness and ignorance of the laws of nature, by spending vast sums

of money, by commissioning research on a gigantic scale, and by propaganda. The attempt will fail, but not before it causes a tremendous explosion in health costs, which, in turn, will lead to serious social upheaval as well as economic and political crises. Even industries that have merged into vast conglomerates in order to finance these nonorthomolecular "medicines" will fail. No amount of money in the world will ever make it possible to imitate the development of effective substances evolved over hundreds of millions of years of biofunctional adaptation, to say nothing of overtaking them. Hans, you are the only medical doctor sitting at this table, but you will see that I shall be proved right.

How right he was! Recently, we have seen evidence that several of the pharmaceutical giants are beginning to feel

Photo taken at the World Congress of the International Academy of Preventative Medicine, Spiring 1974. From left to right: Hans Selye, Mrs. Cohen, Benjamin Cohen, Hans Nieper, Roger Williams, Linus Pauling, and Bob McCullogh (World President Lions Clubs).

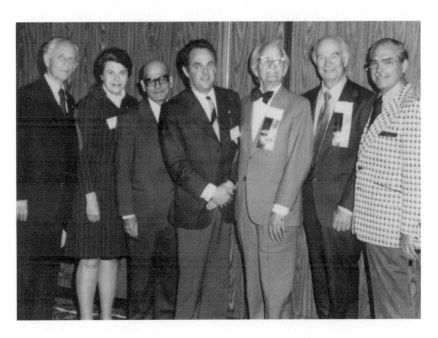

the weight of financial research losses incurred on toxic orthodox substances that simply don't work. For example, Sanyo, a Japanese company in Tokyo, developed a nonorthomolecular substance called Troglitazone. It claimed that Troglitazone improves glucose transport in about 40 percent of type II diabetic patients exhibiting insulin resistance. The product had to be withdrawn from the market by the giant Glaxo-Warner-Lambert conglomerate after about $750 million were spent on marketing Troglitazone because the substance was found to have serious liver-toxicity side effects.

Similarly, Parke-Davis is reported to have lost $400 million to $500 million on other nonorthomolecular developments that have also failed. Hoechst, a German giant in the pharmaceuticals industry, recently laid off its entire pharmaceutical department of 600. In four years, Hoechst spent over 4.5 billion deutschemarks without producing a single new saleable pharmaceutical product. During negotiations with Hoechst several years ago, I predicted this would happen, as I remembered Linus Pauling's words. His foresight was great, indeed.

In addition to his Nobel Prize for biological chemistry, Pauling was awarded the prestigious Nobel Peace Prize for relentless campaigning for the cessation of nuclear testing. He was truly an extraordinary person with great integrity. Pauling's thinking was incredibly clear, direct, and uncomplicated, and his words profoundly influenced me. During my difficult confrontations with various agencies and bureaucracies of the United States government during the 1980s and early 1990s, I often found myself thinking about Linus and his remarks, which have proven so prophetic.

THE SUPERIORITY OF ORTHOMOLECULAR MEDICINE

The first time I heard the term *orthomolecular* was from Linus Pauling, that evening in 1974. I had my doubts as to whether this term would ever gain acceptance. However, to my surprise and to the horror of the orthodox medical establishment, people have learned to understand the term far more quickly than one might have expected. Orthomolecular medicine holds the theory that disease (both mental and physical) is a result of chemical imbalances or deficiencies in the body and can be remedied by restoring proper balance with chemical substances such as vitamins and minerals. Today, the term serves as the foundational definition of many successful alternative therapies.

From Pauling's axiom that *only orthomolecular substances can bring success in long-term therapy*, it follows that only these can achieve a true cure in treating the ravaging effects of such chronic diseases as cancer, decalcification diseases such as osteoporosis, and disorders of the immune system, including the autoimmune diseases of multiple sclerosis, diabetes, and AIDS. Together, these aforementioned diseases represent over 90 percent of all chronic diseases. Nonorthomolecular (toximolecular) substances cannot bring about cures, for they act only as short-term correctives, nor can they bring about any true enhancement of health. At best, toximolecular substances maintain a tolerable balance for a questionable period of time.

It lies in the nature of orthomolecular therapy that its benefits may not become apparent for a number of years— far beyond the normal time allotted by orthodox institutions as a criterion for accepting new therapeutic drugs. Because the evaluation of many orthomolecular therapies can only mature empirically or with time, they will frequently be dismissed by the orthodox school as "unproven," "not recognized," or "not eligible for reimbursement." Unfortunately, the FDA subscribes to instant gratification; a treatment substance must show almost immediate results (in days, not months or years). But orthomolecular medicine aims at attacking the chronic disease at its roots, which often involves genetic reversal. And genetic reversal may take years. Just as many cancers insidiously develop over years, their proper "cures" may take years and/or continuous medication over a long period of time.

MY PROPOSAL FOR THE HEALTHCARE SYSTEM

In the mid-1990s, during President Clinton's first term, the United States Senate experienced a horrendous crisis over the need to cut $740 billion from the healthcare budget. Medical costs have exploded with good reason! Likewise, in Germany and France, the soaring costs of health care have become a permanent challenge. Yet, there has been no radical attempt to overhaul the healthcare systems along the lines suggested by Linus Pauling.

In May, 1992, during the Presidential primaries, I was asked to suggest for Ross Perot guidelines for the reform and treatment of chronic diseases, which include the prevention and treatment of heart and circulatory diseases; calcium deficiency diseases such as osteoporosis; immune-deficiency diseases such as multiple sclerosis; and cancer. I proposed that the treatment of chronic diseases, which account for the great majority of patient visits to health care facilities in the United States, should no longer be based on orthodox, toximolecular, non-biological (synthetic) therapies. When it comes to managing chronic diseases, orthodox medicine has almost totally failed and has caused an explosion in healthcare costs. My proposal for improving national health care includes personal responsibility and the stopping of poisonous pharmaceutical treatments.

Patients must take greater responsibility for their health and well-being. In order to do this, they must be given greater freedom and become better informed about the therapeutic choices available for the prevention and treatment of chronic diseases, particularly information about the advanced orthomolecular therapies. I strive to give patients such information through my tapes, books, lectures, articles, and professional publications.

The essence of my proposal was that orthodox, highly toxic medications from the laboratories of the pharmaceutical industry cease to be used. These medications are prescribed by many cost-insensitive doctors and paid for by private and government medical insurance. The Japanese have recently published several interesting statistics about their healthcare system. The figures indicate that the Japanese incur only about one-third of the German and a quarter of the United States healthcare costs per capita. Furthermore, they live four years longer! The average Japanese life expectancy is 77.4 years, versus U.S. life expectancy of 73.7 years. At their own expense, the Japanese purchase vast quantities of nutrient supplements, such as modern magnesium salts and Glukane from yeasts for cancer prevention. The Japanese represent a huge consumer base, and it is their use of alternative medication that leads to better health care, better prosperity for the individual and the nation's budget, and quite simply, longer life.

The majority of alternative remedies for the prevention and treatment of chronic diseases are of natural (biological) origin or formulation and are nontoxic. Therefore, they could be produced as *nutrient, natural substance,* or *self-treatment remedies,* and could be sold as such. This would make them subject simply to the rules of the free market place, just as foods are. They would become far less expensive than the proprietary toximolecular medications offered by the orthodox medical and pharmaceutical establishment. With the help of good training materials and instruction, consumers could apply these substances, in some cases, to acute illness requiring immediate attention, as well as use them for long-term treatment of serious chronic (degenerative) diseases.

My healthcare proposal eventually landed in the office of Senator Orrin Hatch, a Republican from Utah and a member of the U.S. Senate Committee for Health Reform. It took only a few weeks before Senator Hatch presented my ideas to the Senate. During the summer of 1992, I also presented my proposal at a symposium in New York, where I received a standing ovation. One lady came up to me afterwards and said, "You must present this to Bill Clinton." My plan was shown to Congress shortly after, as several politicians had exposure to its tenets during Perot's campaigning.

The following autumn, Mr. Clinton (not yet President) wrote to Dr. Jonathan Collins, the well-known editor of the *Townsend Letter for Doctors.* In his letter, Mr. Clinton used, word for word, the essence of my healthcare proposal prepared earlier in the year. Following President Clinton's election in 1992, Congressman Bill Richardson, a devoted supporter of and campaign worker for Clinton, subsequently was asked by the President to introduce a bill also embodying some of my proposals for safeguarding and exempting nutrient supplements from overzealous FDA regulations and restrictions. This bill, entitled "The Dietary Supplement Health and Education Act of 1994," was passed by the Congress and signed into law by President Clinton. Thus, the first major step toward acceptance and free access to natural medicine in the U.S. had been taken. People can now "legally" take nutrient supplements to strengthen their bodies and increase their resistance to illness.

My argument promoting natural therapies, many of which could be self-administered, will become a most effective measure to combat spiraling healthcare costs. I was pleased to learn that the Swiss Association of Private Insurance Companies (SWIDA) has since rated natural orthomolecular medicines equal to orthodox medicines for purposes of insurance reimbursement—a principle which has been proposed and hopefully will soon be adopted in Germany, the United States, and other countries.

THE CRISIS OF ORTHODOX MEDICINE

In 1993, Germany's Federal Court of Justice threw a massive "monkey wrench" into the machinations of the orthodox camp by declaring the "Abolition of the Science Clause." This pronouncement places treatments based upon observation, professional and clinical experience, or anecdotal surveys of past precedents on the same footing as those based upon linear, mathematically predictive analysis. The orthodox school had recognized only the latter as a valid basis for the acceptance of new therapies. It will undoubtedly take the proponents of orthodox medicine some years to understand how this ruling will affect them.

Furthermore, the Centrale Marketinggesellschaft der deutschen Agrrarwirtschaft (CMDA), a Bonn (Germany) marketing group, has distributed the publications of Timo Sandberg and other experimental researchers in Helsinki to *all German internists and general practitioners*. Thus, the entire medical community is being exposed to the startling results of the Helsinki study, which determined that a group of heart and circulatory patients treated for more than seven years with orthodox medications (Adalat; Nifedipin; Macumer; beta-blockers; lipid-reducers; nitro-preparations; and diuretics) had more deaths than the group of comparable, untreated participants. (See page 85 for more information on this study.) In principle, these facts have been known for years, but the study put it on paper. In contrast, the nontoxic nutrient supplements—magnesium orotate; bromelain; selenium; serrapeptase; and carnitine—have shown profoundly positive long-term effects on heart vessels and on the conditions of arteriosclerosis and high blood pressure, drastically prolonging life.

In the interim, the Wörwag Company (a manufacturer of magnesium orotate) of Stuttgart, Germany, has published impressive positive data on magnesium orotate's effectiveness on heart and circulatory problems. Their data confirms

that the magnesium orotate penetrates the cellular membranes and enters the interior of the cells, where it can be
very effective in retarding and even reversing heart and
arterial cell damage. My 1968 patent application on the
orotates was based on this concept. At one time, the Heart
Association charged that "these [Nieper] substances are
'unproven' and without value" and demanded that U.S.
Customs intercept and confiscate my patients' medications. Today, the Heart Association is finally endorsing the
therapeutic value of many of these same nutrient supplements that have been used so effectively for decades in
Europe and Japan.

Since the CMDA informed all German internists and general practitioners that conventional heart medications produced more deaths in the long run than those who were
untreated, the orthodox school of medicine has undoubtedly experienced its greatest bankruptcy yet. The entire medical establishment is now attempting damage control
because their orthodox medications have not proved to be
effective in the long-term treatment of chronic diseases.
Some of the large pharmaceutical houses are rethinking
their options regarding nontoxic orthomolecular substances.

Dr. Lichtlen, a well-known German cardiologist, gave a
long interview to a leading medical journal in which he
pointed out that existing surgical and orthodox heart-
attack therapy hardly improves patient life expectancy. Dr.
Lichtlen has had an amazing conversion to this line of
thought, as his earlier medical books hold a very different
opinion. Therefore, time is undoubtedly proving that
orthodox ways are not the best ways.

THE NEED FOR A MORE
ENLIGHTENED PATH OF MEDICINE

It is ironic that among the FDA's list of "unapproved
drugs" sent to my cancer patients in the United States as

recently as 1994 are a number of nutritional supplements, such as carnitine, bromelain, ascorbates, vitamin E, and thymus extract, that are presently readily available over-the-counter (OTC) in most drug and health-food stores in the United States and Europe. How things change! And keep in mind that while the FDA was viciously attacking me and harassing my patients, and while the U.S. Customs department was confiscating the critically needed medications, they made no effort to stop cigarette smoking, proven to cause heart disease and lung cancer. (See "Finding the Truth," on page 160.) It just doesn't seem that the FDA always has the best interest of the people at heart.

Because of the commitment to medical orthodoxy, the costs of health care in the United States have now reached the highest in the world, though the mean life expectancy has fallen to seventeenth place in the world. Since health-care costs and Medicare reserves make up the greater part of the non-wage costs of medical care, these will have to be drastically reduced. The question is, "How?" Amazing cutbacks can be accomplished with sound *preventative* medicine through the broad use of orthomolecular nutritional and dietary supplements.

Our world is in the midst of profound changes—technologically, scientifically, and socially. Many members of the orthodox medical faculty have been blinded by the pharmaceuticals establishment. They see only (bio)chemical phenomena in health and disease; they largely ignore the entirety of the human organism. But without allowing growth and change, there soon will no longer be a place for today's orthodox therapies. If orthodox therapeutic medicine wants to join in our vision of a new biology, it will need to close the gap, which is comparable to abandoning the quill penn for a computer.

I think many medical researchers and practitioners have fallen prey to a disorder that I call "Schoeppensted Syndrome." Schoeppensted is a town in central Germany

Finding the Truth

Recently, in hearings before the U.S. Congress, documents have proven that the tobacco industry lied to the American public about the harmful and addictive properties of nicotine and, therefore, of cigarettes. The Justice Department subsequently obtained a guilty plea from Philip Morris in a criminal case. Numerous state and class-action settlements amounting to billions of dollars have been successfully prosecuted against the tobacco industry, to recover moneys paid for medical care provided to cancer and heart patients. Tobacco-related illness costs the American public over $100 billion annually in medical care and lost wages. Despite these proven facts and legal settlements, there has been no effort to shut down the highly lucrative tobacco industry.

This obvious lack of ethical action on the government's part, when it comes to creating a healthier environment and nation by fighting tobacco use, should trigger a healthy skepticism in government decisions on appropriate health care. I am not saying that Federal government agencies are working for the citizens' ruin, but that many factors slant its decision-making processes and pull it away from better, more responsible decisions. So be wary of buying into what the Federal agencies proclaim about alternative care and the value of nutrient substances. You are not always getting "the truth, and nothing but

where, according to legend, the townspeople constructed the finest, strongest town hall that had ever been seen. They worked tirelessly on the building for months. The foundation was deep, the walls were straight, the roof was watertight, and the doors were square and sturdy. It was only when the town hall was finished that the people realized they had completely forgotten to include windows! The inside of the building was as dark as a tomb. Unwilling to admit their mistake, the people of Schoeppensted tried to illuminate the new town hall by capturing sunlight and bringing it into the building in potato sacks. After days of unsuccessfully dragging in potato sack after potato sack, they gave up, and the building was abandoned. Medical science today—particularly in the United States—is much like the fabled town hall of Schoeppensted, built on a strong foundation but deprived of the light of other sciences and medical traditions.

The problems facing modern medicine in the treatment of chronic illness can only be solved by the use of orthomolecular therapy, which Linus Pauling has bequeathed to us and which I am pledged to provide to my patients. Through this book, I hope I have conveyed to you, my reader, some of this "curious man's" lifelong commitment to treating patients with compassion, to healing them using the most effective orthomolecular therapies available for the prevention and treatment of disease, and to share with you my insights, faith, and confidence in meeting the medical challenges of the future. I believe that, in order to make true progress, science must work for humanity.

Nature talks, just listen.

$\mathcal{S}$ELECTED REFERENCES

Chapter 1: Childhood and the War

Kater, Michael H. *Doctors Under Hitler.* Chapel Hill, North Carolina: The University of North Carolina Press, 1989.

Kurth, Peter. *Anastasia:The Riddle of Anna Anderson.* Boston, Massachusetts: Little, Brown and Company, 1983.

Massie, Robert K. *The Romanovs.* New York, New York: Ballantine Books, 1995.

Chapter 2: Medicine Meets Physics

Becker, Robert O., and Gary Selden. *The Body Electric.* New York, New York: Morrow, 1985.

Clark, Ronald W. *Einstein: The Life and Times.* New York, New York: The World Publishing Company, 1971.

Einstein, Albert. *Ideas and Opinions* (based on *Mein Weltbild*), edited by Carl Seelig et al. New York, New York: The Modern Library, 1994.

Haisch, Bernard, Harold Puthoff, and Alfonso Rueda. "Beyond E = mc^2," The New York Academy of Sciences' *The Sciences* (NovDec 1994): 26–31.

Maier, Lisa A., MD, L.S. Newman, MD, C.S. Rose, MD, MPH. "Sarcoidosis," *The New England Journal of Medicine*, vol 336, no 4 (April 24, 1997): 1224–1234.

Nieper, Hans A., MD. "Autoptische Befund bei Morbus Boeck" (edited in English: "Thesis on Boeck's Sarcoidosis"), *Frankfurter Zeitschrift fur Pathologie*, Bd. 65 (1954): S284–298.

——————. *Conversion of Gravity Field Energy: Revolution in Technology, Medicine, and Society*. Richland Center, Wisconsin: A. Keith Brewer Science Library, 1985.

——————. "Vacuum Field Energy," lecture presented before the Department of Pathology, Hiroshima University, Hiroshima, Japan, March, 1993.

Valone, Thomas. *Electrogravitics Systems*. Washington, D.C.: Integrity Research Institute, 1994.

Chapter 3: Lessons From the Lab

Bannach, P. "In Memoriam Hermann Druckrey," *Journal of Cancer Research Clinical Oncology*, vol 121 (1995): 629–630.

Cowden, W. Lee, MD, W. John Diamond, MD, with Burton Goldberg. *An Alternative Medicine Definitive Guide to Cancer*. Tiburon, California: Future Medicine Publishing, Inc., 1997.

Culbert, Michael L. *Vitamin B₁₇—Forbidden Weapon Against Cancer: The Fight for Laetrile*. New Rochelle, New York: Arlington House Publishers, 1974.

Druckrey, Hermann. "Guest Editorial," *European Journal of Cancer Prevention*, vol 3 (1994): 391–392.

Macdonald, John S. "Hexamethylmelamine: Activity in lymphoma and other tumors," *Cancer Treatment Reviews*, vol 18 (1991): 99–102.

Moss, Ralph W. *Questioning Chemotherapy*. Brooklyn, New

York: Equinox Press, 1995.

Netterberg, Dr. Robert E., and Robert T. Taylor. *The Cancer Conspiracy.* New York, New York: Pinnacle Books, Inc., 1981.

Chapter 4: Nutrient Metabolism and Transport

Cantor, C.R., and P.R. Schimmel. "The Conformation of Macromolecules," *Biophysical Chemistry*, Part 1. New York, New York: W.H. Freeman & Co.

Chappell, D., T.W. Conway, R. Montgomery, A.A. Spector. "Chapter 12: Membranes, Signal Transduction and Eicosanoids," *Biochemistry*, sixth edition. St. Louis, Missouri: University of Iowa College of Medicine, 1996.

Claymore, Charles, Editor-in-Chief. "Chapter 1: Cells, Skin and Epithelium," *The Human Body.* New York, New York: Dorling Kindersley, Ltd., 1995.

Finkelstein, A., and L. Rothfield. "Membrane Biochemistry," *Annual Review of Biochemistry*, vol 37 (1968): 463–491.

Korn, Edward D. "Cell Membranes: Structure and Synthesis." *Annual Review of Biochemistry*, vol 38 (1969): 263–491.

Leonard, J., and J.E. Rothman. "Membrane Asymmetry," *Science*, vol 195 (Feb 1977): 743–753.

Singer, S.J. "The Molecular Organization of Membranes," *University of California at San Diego Department of Biology* (1974): 805–833.

Thomas, Lewis. *The Lives of a Cell: Notes of a Biology Watcher.* New York, New York: The Viking Press, 1974.

Voit, Donald, and Judith Voit. "Chapter 11: Lipids and Membranes," *Biochemistry.* Englewood, New Jersey: John Wiley & Sons, 1990.

Chapter 5: The Mineral Transporters

Blumberger, K., and Hans A. Nieper. "Electrolyte Transport Theory of Cardiovascular Diseases," edited by E. Bajusz and S. Karger, *Electrolytes and Cardiovascular Diseases,* vol 2 (1966): 141–173.

Buist, Robert. "Orotates—Mineral Salts of Vitamin B_{13}" *Biological Applications of Orotates* (1972): 16–25.

Capraro, V., B. Giordana, G.M. Parenti, V.F. Sacchi. "Potassium-dependent amino acid transport in Lapidoptera," *Annals of the New York Acadamy of Sciences,* vol 456 (1985): 248–249.

Chargoff, Erwin, and A.S. Keston. "2-Aminoethylphosphate," *Journal of Biological Chemistry,* vol 134 (1940): 515.

Clayman, Charles, Editor. *The Human Body—Bone Structure and Growth.* New York, New York: Dorling Kindersley, Ltd., 1995:32–37.

Fink, John M. *Third Opinion: An International Directory to Alternative Therapy Centers for the Treatment and Prevention of Cancer and Other Degenerative Diseases.* Garden City Park, New York: Avery Publishing Group, 1988–1997.

Gifford, K.P., H.L. Judd, J. Molton, L.S. Richardson, B.L. Riggs, H.W. Wahner. "Rates of Bone Loss in the Appendicular and Axial Skeletons of Women," *Journal of Clinical Investigation,* vol 77 (1986): 1487–1491.

Kimmich, George A., and Thomas G. Wingrove. "The characterization of intestinal acidic amino acid transport," *Annals of the New York Academy of Sciences,* vol 456 (1985): 80–82.

Merck Research Laboratories. "Osteoporosis," *The Merck Manual,* 16th edition. Whitehouse Station, New Jersey: Merck & Co., Inc., (1992):1357–1359.

Morrisette, George N. "Retrospective Study of the Effect of Calcium 2-AEP (Colamine Phosphate—Vitamin Mi—Membrane Integrity Factor) in Patients with Multiple Sclerosis," presented at the Calcium 2-AEP Conference, 1986. Available through the A. Keith Brewer Science Library, Richland Center, Wisconsin.

Nieper, Hans A. "The anti-inflamatory and immune-inhibiting effects of calcium orotate on bradytrophic tissues," *Agressologie,* vol 10, no 4 (1969): 349–357.

———. "Capillarographic criteria on the effect of magnesium orotate, EPL substances and clofibrate on the elasticity of blood vessels," *Agressologie,* vol 15, no 1 (1974): 73–77.

———. "The clinical applications of lithium orotate, a two year study," *Agressologie,* vol 14, no 6 (1973): 407–411.

———. "A clinical study of calcium transport substances Ca l-dl aspartate and Ca 2-aminoethanol phosphate as potent agents against autoimmunity and other anticytological aggressions," *Agressologie,* vol. VIII, no. 4 (1967): 4–16.

———. "A comparative study of the clinical effect of Ca-l-dl aspartate (calciretard), of Ca 2-aminoethylphosphate (Ca 2-AEP) and of cortisones," *Agressologie,* vol IX, no 3 (1968): 471–474.

———. "The curative effect of a combination of calcium orotate and lithium orotate on primary and secondary chronic (agressive) hepatitis and liver cirrhosis," presented at The Academy of Preventive Medicine, Washington, D.C., March 9, 1974.

———. "Experimental testing of original carcinostatic compounds with potential infracellular activity," *Agressologie,* vol 7, no 3 (1966).

—————————. "Metabolisme du Calcium et du Phosphore des Patients Traites par l'Orotate de Calcium," *Agressologie,* vol 12, no 6 (1971): 401–408.

—————————. *Mineral Transporters.* New York, New York: Grune & Stratton, 1974.

—————————. "The New Vitamin MI (The Membrane Integrity Factor)," *Raum & Zeit* (Aug-Sep 1988): 1–13.

—————————. "Osteoporosis: A New Method of Interpretation & Deep Caesura   in Therapy," *Explore More,* no 19 (1996).

—————————. "Recalcification of bone metastases by calcium diorotate," *Agressologie,* vol 11, no 6 (1970): 495–502.

—————————. "Suppression of Cancer Development by Calcium Colamine Phosphate and by Calcium-l-dl-Aspartate," *Townsend Letter for Doctors & Patients* (Dec 1995): 82.

Chapter 6: Preventing and Treating Cardiovascular Disease

Blumberger, K., and Hans A. Nieper. "Electrolyte Transport Therapy of Cardiovascular Diseases," edited by E. Bajusz and S. Karger. *Electrolytes and Cardiovascular Diseases,* vol 2 (1966): 141–173.

Dickman, Steven. "Mysteries of the Heart," *Discover* (July 1997): 117–119.

Leviton, Richard. "Detoxifying the Heart," *Alternative Medicine Digest,* Issue 20 (1998).

Nieper, Hans A. "Capillarigraphic criteria on the effect of magnesium diorotate, EPL substances and clofibrate on the elasticity of blood vessels," *Agressologie,* vol 15, no 1 (1974): 73–77.

———————. "Silk Worm Enzyme (Serrapeptase) Found Safe, Effective for Carotid Artery Blockage," *Townsend Letters for Doctors & Patients* (April 1997).

Olszewer, Efraim. "Phytotherapeutic Antioxidant Extract for the Treatment of Coronary Insufficiency," *Revista de Oxidologia* (Nov-Dec 1996).

Sinnott, Robert A. "Newly discovered links between herpes viruses and human diseases," *Health Sciences Institute Members Alert* (Feb 1998).

Chapter 7: Detecting and Treating Cancer

Anton, R., C. Bouthan, et al. "Valepotriates: A New Class of Cytotoxic and Antitumor Agents," *Planta Medica*, vol 41 (1981): 21–28.

Ausubel, F.M., B.J. Baker, J.G. Ellis, J.D.G. Jones, and B.J. Staskawiicz. "Molecular Genetics of Plant Disease Resistance," *Science*, vol 268 (1995): 661–667.

Balick, Michael J., and Paul Alan Cox. "The Ethnobotanical Approach to Drug Discovery," *Scientific American* (June 1994): 82–87.

Blaese, R. Michael. "Gene Therapy for Cancer," *Scientific American* (June 1997): 111–115.

Cavill, G.W.K., and D.L. Ford. "The Chemistry of Ants, III. Structure and Reactions of Iridodial," *Australian Journal of Chemistry*, vol 13, no 2 (1960): 296–310.

Cooper, M.D., and H. Weissman. "How the Immune System Develops," *Scientific American* (Sept 1993): 65–71.

Cowden, W. Lee, and W. John Diamond, with Burton Goldberg. *An Alternative Medicine Definitive Guide to Cancer.* Tiburon, California: Future Medicine Publishing, Inc., 1997.

Culbert, Michael L. *Vitamin B_{17}— Forbidden Weapon Against Cancer: The Fight for Laetrile.* New Rochelle, New York: Arlington House Publishers, 1974.

Editorial, "Pharmaceuticals from plants: great potential, few funds," *The Lancet,* vol 343 (June 1994): 1513–1515.

Fitzgerald, George B., and Michael M. Wick. "Antitumor Effects of Biologic Reducing Agents Related to 3,4-Dihydroxybenzylamine: Dihydroxybenzaldehyde, Dihydroxybenzaldoxime, and Dihydroxybenzonitrile," *Journal of Pharmaceutical Sciences,* vol 76, no 7 (July 1987): 513–515.

Hooper, Celia. "Molecular Evolution: Sampling the New Synthesis," *The Journal of NIH Research,* vol 5 (Jan 1993): 66–70.

Isono, N., M., Kochi, N. Niwayama, and K. Shirakabe. "Antitumor Activity of a Benzaldehyde Derivative," *Cancer Treatment Reports,* vol 69, no 5 (May 1985): 533–537.

Kochi, M., Y. Matsumoto, T. Mizuntani, K. Mochizuki, Y. Saito, and S. Takeuchi. "Antitumor Activity of Benzaldehyde," *Cancer Treatment Reports,* vol 64, no 1 (Jan 1980).

Kolberg, Rebecca. "Linking DNA Mismatch Repair to Carcinogenesis," *The Journal of NIH Research,* vol 5 (1993): 32–34.

Ludlow, John W., and Gary R. Skuse. "Tumour Suppressor Genes in Disease and Therapy," *The Lancet,* vol 345 (Apr 1995): 902–906.

Marx, Jean. "How Cells Cycle Towards Cancer," *Science,* vol 263 (1994): 319–321.

————————. "Learning How to Suppress Cancer," *Science: Journal of the New York Academy of Science,* vol 261 (1993): 1385–1387.

————————. "New Link Found Between (Protein) p53

and DNA Repair," *Science,* vol 266 (Nov 1994): 1321–1322.

Nash, J. Madeleine. "The Immortality Enzyme," *Time* (Sept 1, 1997): 65.

Nieper, Hans A. "Experimental testing of original carcinostatic compounds with potential infracellular activity," *Agressologie,* vol VII, no 3 (1966).

—————————. "Genetic Repair, Including 'IRIDODIAL,' an Insect Derived Genetic Repair Factor of Important Antimalignant Effect," *Raum & Zeit* (1990).

—————————. "Iridodial: The Ant Enzyme," *Townsend Letter for Doctors & Patients* (Nov 1997): 84–85.

—————————. "Membrane Repair Against Immune and Degenerative Diseases," lecture presented in Atlanta, Georgia, April 1994. Available through the A. Keith Brewer Science Library, Richland Center, Wisconsin.

—————————. "Modern Medical Cancer Therapy Following the Decline of Toxic Chemotherapy," *Townsend Letter for Doctors & Patients* (Nov 1996): 88.

—————————. "New Developments in Gene Repair," public lecture in Phoenix, Arizona, May 1985. Available through the A. Keith Brewer Science Library, Richland Center, Wisconsin.

—————————. "New Horizons in Non-Toxic Cancer Therapy: Beta Carotene, Lithium Orotate, Anavit, Bromelain, Benzaldehyde, Tumosterone, DHEA, and Ascorbate," *Journal of the International Academy of Preventative Medicine* (Nov 1982): 5–10.

—————————. "The Non-Toxic Long-Term Therapy of Cancer: Necessity State of the Art Trends," *Journal of the International Academy of Preventive Medicine,* vol VI, no1 (1980): 42–70.

—————————. "Recalcification of bone metastases by Calcium Diorotate," *Agressologie*, vol XI, no 6 (1970): 495–502.

—————————. "Suppression of Cancer Development by Calcium Colamine Phosphate and by Calcium-l-dl-Aspartate," *Townsend Letter for Doctors & Patients* (Dec 1996): 82.

—————————. "The Treatment of Malignant Processes with Substances of Potential Genetic Repair Effect, Recent Advances and Developments," presented at The World Cancer Congress, Sydney, Australia, April 1994.

Richards, Dick. *The Topic of Cancer.* London, England: Pergamon House, 1982.

Rosenthal, Nadia. "Regulation of Gene Expression," *Molecular Medicine*, vol 331, no 14 (1994): 931–933.

Service, Robert. "Slow DNA Repair Implicated in Mutations Found in Tumors," *Science*, vol 261 (Mar 1994): 1374.

Thies, P.W. "Iridoide und andere terpenoid Naturstoffe," *Pharmazie in unserer Zeit*, vol XIV, no 2 (1985): 33–40.

Travis, John. "Tracing the Immune System's Evolutionary History," *Science*, vol 261 (July 1993): 164–165.

von Hippel, Peter H. "Protein-DNA Recognition: New Perspectives and Underlying Themes," *Science*, vol 263 (Feb 1994): 769–770.

Walker, Morton. "Venus Flytrap: Cancer and AIDS Fighter of the Future?" *East West Natural Health*, vol 22, no 5 (1992).

—————————. "The Carnivora Cure for Cancer, AIDS, and Other Pathologies," *Townsend Letter for Doctors & Patients* (June 1991): 412–416.

Yoon, Carol Kaesuk. "Nibbled Plants Don't Just Sit There;

They Launch Active Attacks," *The New York Times,* section C (June 23, 1992): 1, 12.

Chapter 8: *Understanding and Treating Multiple Sclerosis*

Chargoff, Erwin, and A.S. Keston. "2-Aminoethyl-phosphate," *Journal of Biological Chemistry,* vol 134 (1940): 515.

Morrisette, George N. "Retrospective Study of the Effect of Calcium 2-AEP (Colamine Phosphate—Vitamin M_i—Membrane Integrity Factor) in Patients with Multiple Sclerosis," presented at the Calcium 2-AEP Conference, 1986. Available through the A. Keith Brewer Science Library, Richland Center, Wisconsin.

Morrissette, Claire V. *Hope for Us! Taking Positive Action Against Multiple Sclerosis with the CaAEP Treatment and Necessary Lifestyle Changes.* Augusta, Maine: Gannett Graphics, 1985.

Nieper, Hans A. "A Clinical Study of Calcium Transport Substances Ca-*l-dl*-Aspartate and Ca-2-Aminoethylphosphate as Potent Agents Against Auto-immunity and Other Anticytological Aggressions," *Agressologie,* vol VIII, no.4 (1967): 4–16.

————. "A Comparative Study of the Clinical Effect of Ca-*l-dl*-Aspartate (Calciretard), of Ca-2-Aminoethylphosphate (Ca-2-AEP) and of Cortisones," *Agressologie,* vol IX, no 3 (1968): 471–474.

————. "Membrane Repair Against Immune and Degenerative Diseases," presented in Atlanta, Georgia, April 1994. Available through the A. Keith Brewer Science Library, Richland Center, Wisconsin.

————. "Metabolisme du Calcium et du Phosphore des Pateints Traites par l'Orotate de Calcium," *Agressologie,* vol XII, no 6 (1971): 401–408.

——————. "The New Vitamin Mi (The Membrane Integrity Factor)," *Raum & Zeit* (Aug-Sep 1988): 1–13.

Chapter 9: Fame and Infamy

Altman, Lawrence K. "Experts See Bias in Drug Data, Tied to Research Sponsorship," *The New York Times* (April 29, 1997).

Bandow, Doug. "The FDA Can Be Dangerous to Your Health," *Fortune* (Nov 11, 1996): 56.

Congressional Record. "West German Cancer Specialist Visits the United States," Congressions Record, Extension of Remarks, March 31, 1980.

Cowden, W. Lee, and W. John Diamond, with Burton Goldberg. *An Alternative Medicine Definitive Guide to Cancer.* Tiburon, California: Future Medicine Publishing, Inc., 1997.

Culbert, Michael L. *Vitamin B₁₇— Forbidden Weapon Against Cancer: The Fight for Laetrile.* New Rochelle, New York: Arlington House Publishers, 1974.

Dumoff, Alan. "Expanding the OAM (NIH Office of Alternative Medicine) Into a Center for Integral Medicine and Creating Access to Medical Treatment," *Alternative & Complementary Therapies* (Feb 1997): 59–63, and Appendix, 1–13.

Miller, Monica. "The Health Freedom Movement in the States," *FAIM (Foundation for the Advancement of Innovative Medicine) Innovation,* no 2 (1997).

Moss, Ralph W. *Questioning Chemotherapy.* Brooklyn, New York: Equinox Press, 1995.

Netterberg, Dr. Robert E., and Robert T. Taylor. *The Cancer Conspiracy.* New York, New York: Pinnacle Books, Inc., 1981.

Patton Boggs, L.L.P. *The Dietary Supplement Health and Education Act of 1994: Section-by-Section Overview and Analysis.* Washington, D.C. (1994): 1–26, and Appendices including Statement by President William J. Clinton on signing Senate Bill *S. 784.*

Thomas, Lewis. *The Lives of a Cell: Notes of a Biology Watcher.* New York, New York: The Viking Press, 1974.

United States Food and Drug Administration. *FDA Regulation Report,* vol II, no 3 (Mar 1997).

——————. *FDA Regulation Report,* vol II, no 7 (July 1997).

Chapter 10: A More Reasoned Approach

Astrow, Alan B. "Rethinking Cancer," *The Lancet,* vol 343 (1994): 494–495.

Beardsley, Tim. "A War Not Won: Trends in Cancer Epidemiology," *Scientific American* (Jan 1994): 130–138.

Bergner, Paul. "German Evaluation of Herbal Medicines," *The Journal of the American Botanical Council and the Herb Research Foundation, HerbalGram,* no 30 (1994): 17.

Buckley, Nicholas A. "Evidence-based Medicine in Toxicology: Where is the Evidence?" *The Lancet,* vol 347 (1996): 1067–1069.

Brown, Chip. "The Experiments of Dr. Oz," *The New York Times Magazine* (July 30, 1995): 20–23.

Herman, Joseph. "Experiment and Observation," *The Lancet,* vol 344 (Oct 29, 1994): 1209–1210.

Lammi, Glenn. "Should Congress Curb the FDA's Power over Drugs, Vitamins, and Medical Devices?" *Health* (May/June 1995): 34.

Nieper, Hans A. "The Crisis of Mechanistic Medicine and

the Progress of Eumetabolic Preventive and Protective Medicine," presented before the International Academy of Preventive Medicine, Houston, Texas, 1978.

――――――――. "The Crisis of Orthodox Medicine is Gaining Momentum," *Raum & Zeit* (May/June 1993): 1–8.

――――――――. "Linus Pauling and Orthomolecular Medicine," *Health & Healing*, Australia, vol 16, no 4 (Aug/Oct 1997): 18–22.

Rhein, Reginald. "Sound and Fury or Real Reform at FDA?" *The Journal of NIH Research,*vol 7 (May 1995): 26–27.

Rothman, Kenneth. "Use of Placebo Controls in Clinical Trials Disputed," *Science,* vol 267 (Jan 6, 1995): 25–26.

Taubes, Gary. "Looking for the Evidence in Medicine," *Science,* vol 272 (Apr 5, 1996): 22–24.

Tyler, Varro E. *Natural Products and Medicine—An Overview.* West Lafayette, Indiana: School of Pharmacy and Pharmacal Sciences, Purdue University. Reprinted by *HerbalGram,* no 28 (1993): 40–41.

$\mathcal{S}$UGGESTED READINGS

Culbert, Michael L. *Vitamin B_{17}—Forbidden Weapon Against Cancer: The Fight for Laetrile.* New Rochelle, New York: Arlington House Publishers, 1974.

Lopez, D.A., MD, M. Miehlke, MD, R.M. Williams, MD, PhD, *Enzymes: The Fountain of Life.* Charleston, South Carolina: The Neville Press, Inc., 1994.

Moss, Ralph W. *Questioning Chemotherapy: A Critique of the Use of Toxic Drugs in the Treatment of Cancer.* Brooklyn, New York: Equinox Press, 1995.

Moss, Ralph W. *The Cancer Industry: The Classic Expose on the Cancer Establishment.* Revised ed. Brooklyn, New York: Equinox Press, 1996.

Nieper, Hans A., MD. "Suppression of Cancer Development by Calcium Colamine Phosphate and by Calcium-l-dl-Aspartate," *Townsend Letter for Doctors & Patients.* December (1996): 82.

Pallares, Demetrio Sodi, MD. *Lo Que He Descubierto en el Tejido Canceroso: Tratamiento Metabólico Para Enfermos Cancerosos Desahuciados.* Mexico: 1998.

About 400 of Dr. Hans Nieper's medical papers, and about 300 space physics papers, in addition to his books and brochures, are on file in the Hans Nieper, MD, archives at:

The A. Keith Brewer International Science Library
325 North Central Avenue
Richland Center, WI 53581
Telephone: 608-647-6513
Fax: 608-647-6797
Email: drbrewer@mwt.net
Web site: http://www.mwt.net/~drbrewer

$\mathcal{A}$BOUT THE AUTHORS

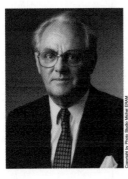

Hans A. Nieper, MD, is world-renowned for his treatment of cancer, multiple sclerosis, bone disorders, aging, diabetes, kidney disorders, and cardiac disease. He has developed a number of effective, orthomolecular substances over the course of his career. As an Internist, Dr. Nieper practices in West Germany, successfully treating a large number of patients from all over the world. Furthermore, approximately 360 of Dr. Nieper's articles and essays are published, and he has appeared on over a dozen radio and television programs and lectured extensively throughout the United States and the world.

In advancing medical science, Dr. Nieper has taken an inter-disciplinary approach. His work in physics, including his widely respected "Shielding Theory of Gravity," led to his conviction that there is an inextricable relationship between the energy of the universe, the body's cellular energy, and each individual's personal health. His book, *Dr. Nieper's Revolution in Technology and Medicine,* explores this concept.

Dr. Nieper is a life member of the German Society of Natural Scientists and Physicians, and was the President of the German Society of Oncology from 1983 to 1987. He is the founder and Past President of the German Association of Vacuum Field Energy, a member of France's Society Agressologie, the New York Academy of Sciences, and the American Association for the Advancement of Science, and also served for two years as Honorary President of the International Academy of Preventative Medicine.

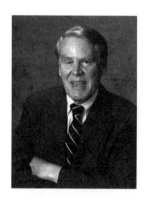

Arthur Douglass Alexander graduated from Case Institute of Technology, where he majored in chemical engineering and engineering management. Later, he completed graduate studies in biochemistry at Cornell Medical College (Sloan-Kettering Biosciences Division). Alexander has over thirty-five years experience in chemical and biological research and management activities. He served as assistant to Dr. C. Chester Stock, Scientific Director of the Sloan-Kettering Institute for Cancer Research in New York, where he met Dr. Nieper. They became life-long friends.

Alexander was then appointed Associate Director of the Children's Cancer Research Foundation in Boston. Next, he worked with Dr. Edwin Land on the development of Polaroid color film with the Polaroid Corporation, followed by a position as a Senior Scientist with NASA. For fifteen years, Alexander was an adviser in immunological research to the late Dr. Virginia Livingston, and served on the Board of Directors of the Livingston Foundation of San Diego.

Alexander continues to pursue his long-standing interest in immunology, cancer research, and space physics. He is a member of many professional associations, including the New York Academy of Sciences, the American Chemical Society, and the Royal Society of Chemists. In addition, Alexander is a Fellow of the American Institute of Chemists. He has authored numerous papers and publications. A retired biochemist and research scientist, Alexander currently works as a scientific consultant and writer, and lives with his wife, Virginia, in Sonoma, California.

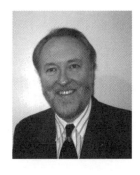

Gene Sylvester Eagle-Oden graduated from Mineral Area College and the University of Missouri with degrees in electrical engineering, management, and market research, and began an interesting and varied career in several fields. In computer sciences, he was active in Control Data's support of the Simulation Laboratory during NASA's Apollo moon probe project. Later, Honeywell Corporation named him "New Marketing Director of the World" for his work on automating the St. Louis and Chicago commodities exchanges, and for implementing a computerized program for the production of steel pipe components from recycled metal. By age thirty, Mr. Oden was recognized in "Who's Who in American-Equipment Leasing" for financial excellence and he also began an active tax and financial services practice which led to the facilities management of two 500-bed hospitals.

However, within a few years, Mr. Oden decided to sell his businesses and dedicate himself to a new life's direction—"helping the people of the world achieve their dreams through better health." Since meeting Dr. Hans Nieper in 1985, Mr. Oden has fully devoted his resources and energy to promoting complementary and natural medical alternative methodologies and products, especially those of Dr. Nieper. In 1994, he founded the Health Freedom Foundation and became an active lobbyist, domestically and internationally. He attended the world assembly, *Codex Alimentarius*, in Bonn in 1996 and Berlin in 1998.

Currently, Mr. Eagle-Oden officially represents the New Zealand Charter of Health Practitioners, as well as other organizations. In addition, he is cofounder and President and Managing Director of the International Federation of Health Practitioner Associations, which represents the interests of many complementary and biological healthcare associations worldwide.

*𝓘*NDEX

substances that affect, 52–53
types of. *See* Arginates;
Aspartates; Orotates;
2-aminoethylphosphate.
Mitochondria, 48, 49
Mitochondrial organelles. *See*
Mitochondria.
Moenninghoff, Dr., 63
Morrisette, Dr. George, 63, 129
Moss, Dr. Ralph, 40–41, 141
MS. *See* Multiple sclerosis.
Multiple sclerosis (MS), 115–117,
119–121
blood-brain-barrier (BBB)
type, 118–119
conventional therapies for,
124–125
possible causes of, 121–124
squalene and, 128
treatment program for,
125–129
2-AEP salts and, 63–64,
126–127
Myelin sheath, 116, 117, 119,
120, 123

National Cancer Institute (NCI),
35, 39, 40, 104, 142
National Health Foundation, 144
NCI. *See* National Cancer
Institute.
New England Journal of Medicine, 29
Nieper, Dr. Hans A., early histo-
ry of, 6–9, 11–19, 24–30
Nitrilosides, 37–38
Nitrogen mustards, 32
Nucleus, 48, 49
Nuremberg race laws, 10–11
Nutrients
breakdown of, 45–47
transport of, 49–50. *See also*
Mineral transporters.

OAM. *See* Office of Alternative
Medicine.

Oberling, Dr., 84
Office of Alternative Medicine
(OAM), 145
Old, Dr. Lloyd, 35
Oligodendroglia. *See* Medullary
sheath.
Oncostatins, 108
Orotates, 58–60
Orthomolecular medicine,
about, 152–154
Ozone treatment, 73–74

Passive diffusion, 50
Paul Ehrlich Institute of
Experimental Therapy,
33–34
Pauling, Dr. Linus, 132, 150,
152–153, 154
Perisolar cushion field theory,
22
P-53 protein, 84
Physics, about, 24
Plant extract. *See* Carnivorous
plant extract.
Plumbagin, 105
Potassium orotate, 59–60
Potassium-magnesium
aspartate, 53, 56–57, 79–80

Questioning Chemotherapy
(Moss), 41, 141

Radiation therapy, 94–95
Raum und Zeit, 60
Relativity, Einstein's Theory of,
20
Retrovir, 112
Rhodanase, 38
Ribosomes, 48, 49

Sarcoidosis, 29
Schrauzer, Prof. G., 81
Schwartz, Dr. Arthur, 106
Sciences, The, 23
Selenium, 80

deficiency of, 83–84
Selye, Dr. Hans, 47, 52, 79, 150
Serrapeptase, 81–82
Shark liver oil. *See* Squalene.
Shielding Theory of Gravity,
    20–23
Sills, Dr. Allen K., 110
Sinnott, Dr. Robert A., 83
Squalene, 109–110, 128
Sloan-Kettering Institute for
    Cancer Research, 34–35, 39,
    40, 141
Statin therapy, 72
Stock, Dr. C. Chester, 35, 41
Streptokinase, 75
Stress, cancer and, 91–92
Stroke, 74
Sugiura, Dr., 39, 40
Surgery
    arteriosclerosis and, 71
    cancer and, 92–93

Takeuchi, Setsuo, 104
Taussig, Dr. Steven, 73
Thalidomide, 135–136, 139–140
Thies, Dr. Peter, 107
Third Reich, medical policies of,
    10–11
Thrombosis, 74
    alternative therapy for, 75
    conventional therapy for,
    74–75
Tobacco industry, 160
Todaro, Dr., 108
Townsend Letter for Doctors, 60, 156
Tripertenoid, 128

Troglitazone, 152
Trophosphamide, 124
Tumosterons, 110–111
2-AEP. *See* 2-aminoethyl-
    phosphate.
2-AEP complex, 65–67, 83
2-aminoethylphosphate
    (2-AEP), 62–67, 83, 129

Ureyl-mandelonitrile. *See*
    Mandelonitrile.

Vacuum field, 24–28, 117, 119
Vacuoles, 48, 49
Vesicle sacs. *See* Vesicles.
Vesicles, 48, 49
Viruses
    chronic disease and, 83–85
    multiple sclerosis and,
    123–124
    See also Herpes simplex virus.
Vitamin B_{17}. *See* Laetrile.
*Vitamin B_{17}—Forbidden Weapon
    Against Cancer* (Culbert),
    132
Voltage-dependent channels.
    See Ion channels.
Von Nida, Dr. S., 53, 79

Wildenthal, Dr. Kern, 75–76, 77
World War II, effects of, 9–16

Zero point field (ZPF), 23
Zinc arginate, 61–62
Zinc aspartate, 57
ZPF. *See* Zero point field.